Ask the Vet

Ask the Vet

Dawn Curie Thomas, DVM
and William S. Thomas

BookWorld Press and BRIIA

Published by BookWorld Press and BRIIA

Distributed by
BookWorld Services, Inc.
1933 Whitfield Park Loop
Sarasota, FL 34243
24 hour order line: 1-800-444-2524

Publisher's Cataloging in Publication

Thomas, Dawn Curie
Ask the vet / Dawn Curie Thomas and
William S. Thomas. —2nd ed.
    p. cm.
    Includes index.
    ISBN: 1-884962-06-8

    1. Veterinary medicine. 2. Pets—Miscellanea. I. Thomas,
William S. (William Sherman) II. Title.

SF751.T46   636.089

This book is dedicated to all of the ill, injured, neglected and abused little animals that we have taken into our home and into our veterinary hospital and into our hearts over the years, including dear Zonkers, Winston the squirrel, and all of our wonderful cats—Cosette and Eponine, Banana, Bonzal and even grumpy ol' Ouiser.

Table of Contents

Introduction

I am a veterinarian who dearly loves animals and wants them to have the very best possible care.

During my years of veterinary practice, pet owners have asked me thousands of questions about their dogs and cats. This book is a collection of the most commonly asked questions and the answers.

While I can't offer a specific diagnosis for your own pet without actually doing a physical examination, the information in this book will make you more aware of the typical symptoms and usual treatments of these most common problems.

I tend to favor a more "natural" approach than some other veterinarians. For example, I encourage an emphasis on proper nutrition, high-quality skin care products and certain vitamin supplements, because I have observed their dramatic benefits over the years. I always try to avoid treatments that use harsh chemicals or potentially dangerous steroids.

However, I also believe that it is very important to be aggressive with medicine and surgery when appropriate, and always insist on full workups including laboratory tests when your pet is ill.

Our pets are very special to us. They deserve the best health care possible.

— Dawn Curie Thomas, DVM

Abscesses

Q: My big, macho tomcat lost a fight last week. Most of his wounds healed quickly, but one of them is still swollen and sore. What should I do?

A: Your cat probably has developed an abscess. The skin of a cat usually heals so rapidly after a wound that bacteria can become trapped in the tissues, resulting in an infected pocket of pus. The skin may appear red, hot and swollen, and the area around the abscess may be painful. Often cats with abscesses become depressed and lose their appetites. They might also try to hide from their owners.

Some of the most common causes of abscesses are bite wounds or other lacerations from fights. Abscesses may be located on any part of the body that has been wounded, especially the face, legs and base of the tail.

If your cat develops an abscess you should take your cat to a veterinarian immediately. Shaving the area will reveal the degree of tissue damage; puncture wounds or lacerations may also become obvious for the first time. Usually it is necessary to lance the abscess to flush and drain the wound. Often a tube is inserted to allow drainage of the pus. Antibiotics will be needed to fight the infection. Your veterinarian might have you flush the wound at home with an antibacterial solution or apply warm compresses to aid healing.

As deadly viruses can be transmitted through bite wounds, while your cat is at the veterinary clinic, it would be wise to have him tested for the feline leukemia virus (FeLV) and feline AIDS (FIV), and receive any appropriate vaccinations.

In addition, you should consider having your cat neutered, which probably would make him less interested in roaming and fighting.

Acne

Q: My cat gets horrible pimples and boils on her chin, and sometimes they get red and swollen. What could be causing that?

A: Some cats, like humans, have a tendency to develop acne when excessive oils and dirt accumulate deep in the pores of the skin on the chin or lower lip.

Cat owners may observe blackheads, and the skin can look red, swollen and irritated. If left untreated, blackheads often progress to become papules and pimples. Feline acne, which is seen in mature cats as well as adolescents, usually doesn't bother the cat unless a bacterial infection causes pimples or open sores with draining pus and crusty areas. The hair in these areas often will fall out, leaving bald patches.

In severe cases of acne, your veterinarian may discover that your cat has a fever and swollen lymph nodes. Skin scrapings will be necessary to rule out mites, and a sample of the pus may be needed to culture the bacteria so proper antibiotics can be prescribed. A fungal culture also is recommended to rule out infections such as ringworm.

Treatment of feline acne also usually includes gentle cleansing and warm compresses on the area with a medicated gel applied afterward. Extreme care must be taken to avoid scarring. Never rub, but gently pat when applying the medication.

In severe cases, a cat may have to be sedated so the hair can be clipped from the area and the blackheads removed. Oral antibiotics may have to be used. Acne can be easily controlled, but cats with this problem usually need to continue indefinitely with the preventive treatments.

Foods and supplements such as kelp that contain high concentrations of iodine should be avoided because they can make the acne worse.

Aggressive Dogs

Q: My husband wants to get a pit bull puppy, but I'm worried because we have a two-year-old child. Aren't pit bulls dangerous?

A: Pit bull terriers may have a genetic tendency to want to fight other dogs, but usually their aggressiveness is primarily the result of encouragement from their owners.

In general, any dog's behavior is determined by several factors, including genetic makeup, environment and training.

Pit bulls can be very sweet, devoted pets. However, their genetic history makes it a good practice to take extra precautions when they are around other dogs or even small children.

Every animal should be judged on an individual basis. Dogs are pack animals, and males in particular naturally want to be the top dog or leader of the pack. Therefore, it is critical that human family members are dominant instead.

Breeds that have a reputation for sometimes being aggressive without warning include Akitas, Chow Chows, Rottweilers and Shar-Peis.

AIDS Patients With Pets

Q: My son has AIDS and has moved back home with us. Do you think we should get a dog or a cat to help cheer him up?

A: Dogs and cats can be very emotionally therapeutic for AIDS patients; they can help lower blood pressure, reverse depression and even improving the immune system. And pets don't make judgments.

Since AIDS patients have a suppressed immune system and are more susceptible to a variety of infections, it is important for your son to consult his physician and work closely with a veterinarian to choose a healthy animal to minimize any risk.

For example, toxoplasmosis is a parasite that can be transmitted to humans through the stool of infected cats. In the past, the main concern was the exposure of pregnant women and potential harm to the unborn child, but people with any kind of immune deficiency should also take special precautions against this infection. Roundworms and giardia are other parasites that can also cause problems for AIDS victims.

Skin infections, such as ringworm or scabies, also can be passed from dogs and cats to humans. People who have AIDS are particularly susceptible.

Salmonella and campylobacter are bacteria that can be carried in the stool of dogs and cats and are a source of intestinal infection. Symptoms include a loose stool or diarrhea.

Any pets that come in contact with your son or people that share the same house should have a complete physical exam by a veterinarian every six months.

Outside cats should be tested for toxoplasmosis twice each year, and a combination feline AIDS test and a feline leukemia virus (FeLV) test should be given annually.

AIDS patients should not clean litter boxes or come in contact with loose stools or diarrhea.

Allergic to Your Own Pet?

Q: My boyfriend is allergic to my cats, but I can't decide who to give up—them or him. Any suggestions?

A: People who are allergic to cats are actually reacting to a protein that builds up on the cat's skin. Researchers have found that giving your cats regular baths can help solve the problem.

The protein, called Fel d1, can cause people to sneeze. It is produced both by glands in a cat's skin and by the cat's saliva glands. As the cat licks its fur, it adds to the irritating protein buildup in its dander.

Most cats don't get bathed as regularly as dogs, so the allergens that cause your boyfriend to sneeze keep building up on your cats' skin week after week. If you bathe your cats every month with an appropriate hypoallergenic shampoo, the problem should virtually disappear.

The research on this problem was done at a leading medical school, where allergists were attempting to prove that vitamin A derivatives might shut down the skin gland activity and help solve the problem of allergic reactions to cats. During the study, they gave some cats the vitamin A derivatives and some cats a placebo.

To gauge the amount of the Fel d1 protein left in the cats' dander, the researchers washed each cat monthly during the study, and measured how much of the allergen ended up in the bath water. After eight months, they could barely find any of the protein—on any of the cats. Since even the cats that were getting placebos instead of vitamin A derivatives were free of the protein, researchers concluded that it was the bathing that was getting rid of the problem.

Some cats dislike water, so you may want to have your cat bathed at a veterinary clinic or at a grooming parlor. Make sure the hypoallergenic shampoo that is used is free of chemicals and harsh agents that can strip the hair coat and irritate the skin. (See *Skin Care Products*.)

If you decide to bathe your cat at home, brush out your pet's coat completely before bathing. Always stroke and talk to your pet before and during the bath to help keep your special friend calm and reassured.

Cat dander is sticky and clings to walls and carpets for months, so it is a good idea to thoroughly clean your house after you bathe your cats.

All the Right Stuff

Q: I've adopted a stray dog and want to be sure that he gets all the right stuff. What should I buy for him at the pet store to get started?

A: Walk into any pet store and you will be amazed

at the number and variety of pet supplies—from basics like food and collars to wonderful extras like high-tech electronic devices to keep your dog from roaming or chic, jeweled fashions complete with sweaters and matching hats.

Start with the basics. Always buy premium dog food because nutrition is the basis for good health.

Every pet should have a comfortable, good quality collar and an ID tag with the animal's name, address and telephone number. A rabies tag usually is required by law. Your dog also should have a leash for outdoor activities and travel.

Separate food and water bowls are necessary. The styles vary considerably—from stainless steel or ceramic to plastic. Plastic bowls are cheaper but sometimes get chewed. Heavy bowls won't slide around when your pet eats. Some bowls feature designs to keep ants out of the food.

Get a good book, video or sign up for a class on how to train your dog. A well-behaved pet can be a joy, and a pet that has behavior problems can cause misery for everyone. Usually a few simple tips can help you teach manners and discipline. Routine dental care at home is very important for pets. Get your dog a special toothbrush and non-foaming toothpaste available at pet stores or veterinary clinics. Use them regularly. Also, buy a chew toy that will not only entertain your dog but will help keep tartar off the teeth. Some chew toys work like dental floss to clean between the teeth.

Other play toys are important to keep your dog

active and entertained, and to prevent such destructive "play" as chewing your shoes or roughing up your furniture.

Grooming aids are necessary to keep your pet looking its best. Get a brush that is appropriate for your dog's hair coat, a flea comb and high-quality skin care products. (See *Skin Care Products*.)

Provide your pet with a bed of blankets or perhaps the fancier simulation sheep skins. Dogs that have to sleep on concrete or hard ground sometimes develop contact allergies or sores.

Pet store staffs can give you additional suggestions and tell you about the newest in pet supplies.

Anal Glands

Q: My little dog spends a lot of time scooting around on the floor on his rear end and then licking that area. What could cause such behavior?

A: The "scooting" you describe often is a result of impacted anal glands. The discomfort that your dog feels is temporarily relieved and soothed by licking the area or rubbing it against something—usually the floor.

Anal sacs, or glands, are small pouches located on both sides of the anus of a cat or a dog. These sacs are filled with a brown, watery, foul-smelling secretion that is believed to have been used by wild animals to mark their territory. The anal glands have no known useful function in modern domesticated pets.

Normally, anal glands are emptied when a dog or cat has a bowel movement. Occasionally the sacs are suddenly expressed when an animal is frightened or stressed. This can be a particularly unpleasant experience because of the obnoxious odor.

Medical problems with the anal glands can occur when the glands become full or the ducts inside the sacs become clogged. The result is an impacted anal gland. This causes the dog or cat a great deal of discomfort, and the pet will scoot or lick itself in an attempt to get some relief.

Sometimes an impacted anal gland becomes infected, forming a large, swollen, bloody, pus-filled abscess that should be treated by a veterinarian.

Periodic expression of anal glands is important to keep them from becoming infected or abscessed. Most veterinarians recommend routine manual expression of the anal glands. This unpleasant job can be done by a veterinarian, animal health technician, groomer or someone who is trained in doing the procedure. However, improper emptying of the anal glands can force matter deeper into the tissues and cause additional problems.

If anal glands are severely impacted or infected, a veterinarian may find it necessary to anesthetize your pet to thoroughly empty the anal sacs and infuse them with medication.

In some chronic cases, the anal glands should be

surgically removed.

Anesthesia

Q: Is it true that the anesthesia procedure is the riskiest part of surgery? How safe are anesthetics used in veterinary medicine?

A: Tremendous advances have been made in the use of anesthesia during the last decade that greatly increase safety during surgery. Many of the anesthetics used in veterinary medicine are the same as those that are used in human medicine.

More pets probably die each year from health problems that aren't corrected surgically because of fear of anesthesia than those that die as a result of the dangers of anesthesia itself.

A pre-anesthetic workup is critical before any surgery. This consists of a thorough physical by a veterinarian and often includes a blood test and urinalysis. In some cases, X-rays and an electro-cardiogram are recommended.

These tests are necessary to make sure there aren't underlying medical problems such as kidney or liver disease, diabetes or chronic infection that would put the patient at greater risk during surgery. Also, the tests help the surgeon determine the best type of anesthetic procedure to use.

The rule of thumb is that the older the pet and the more severe the problem, the more thorough the pre-anesthesia workup should be. Proper monitoring of anesthesia helps to improve safety during surgery.

Many veterinary clinics have an EKG or heart monitor which constantly checks the heart rate of the patient and warns the surgeon if there is a problem. Also, trained veterinary technicians usually help the surgeon monitor the pet's respiration, color, eye reflexes and the level of anesthesia.

Gas anesthesia is generally considered to be safer than injectable anesthesia for most surgical procedures, since the gas levels can be increased or decreased quickly as needed.

One of the newest anesthesias available today is isoflurane. This gas provides a high degree of safety with very low toxicity. Isoflurane doesn't alter the patient's heart rate or blood pressure, and the pet wakes up very rapidly after surgery. This gas is an ideal anesthetic for older pets or surgery patients that have other medical problems such as heart, liver or kidney disease.

Another Cat?

Q: I have a two-year-old female cat that seems lonely because I am away at work most of the time. If I get another kitty to keep her company, will it cause problems?

A: Depending on your cat's personality, getting a new kitty could be a great idea or might be entirely unwelcome. Some cats are more social and will interact with the newcomer, while others thrive on getting all of the attention.

A female with a mellow personality probably would be the best choice as your second cat.

Before exposing your lonely cat to her new roommate, take the new cat to a veterinarian for a complete physical exam.

Make sure the newcomer is negative for the feline leukemia virus (FeLV) and the deadly feline AIDS (FIV). She should get vaccinations for feline distemper (FVR-CP), feline leukemia, feline infectious peritonitis (FIP) and rabies. The veterinarian also will examine her teeth, check her for worms and determine if she has been spayed.

Only after you are sure the newcomer is healthy should you bring her home. Of course, this would be a good time to have a physical exam for your two-year-old cat to make sure she is healthy, too.

Introducing the new cat to the household can be a pleasure for you, for her and for your lonely cat, but it should be done carefully for best results. If the newcomer has a contagious disease, you will never forgive yourself for exposing your healthy cat. And, if the cats are suddenly forced to share the same living quarters, they might not get along.

It is best to introduce the cats slowly. Their first choice is not to have other cats in their territory. Often there will be some hissing and other aggressive behavior for several days or weeks.

Begin by putting the new cat in one room of the house with her litter, water and food. Allow the first contact with your lonely cat to be a paw under the door, then after awhile open the door slightly.

Sometimes a little catnip can help cats relax as they get acquainted, much like some people use a social drink at a party. Supervise the interaction between your two cats as much as possible, and try to limit their time together to short periods during the first few days.

After about a week, start feeding them in the same room so that being together will be a positive experience. You can keep one cat in a cage while she is eating and place the other cat's bowl just outside the cage. That will force them to eat face-to-face and accept each other more rapidly.

Provide each cat with an individual litter box to prevent a protest that might take the form of accidents on your carpet.

Arthritis

Q: My twelve-year-old German shepherd has arthritis in her legs and hips. She is starting to get pretty uncomfortable and has trouble getting around. What do you suggest?

A: Older dogs often suffer from arthritis, an inflammation of the joints in the hips, lower back, shoulders and knees. A variety of treatments are available that can make your pet more comfortable.

Joints tend to stiffen when they are not used for

long periods of time, but become less uncomfortable as they warm up from moving. Painful, swollen, stiff joints and the resulting lameness is caused by degeneration of the cartilage. Cracks and erosion develop from injuries, autoimmune disease, and simple wear and tear due to age. Hip displasia and out-of-joint knees also are common causes of arthritis.

Your veterinarian probably will recommend X-rays to determine the cause and location of the diseases that might be causing the lameness.

If your dog is overweight, the first step of treatment usually is a simple reducing diet. This decreases the work load on the affected joints.

Light exercise should continue on a regular basis. For example, daily short walks on a leash over level ground would be appropriate if your pet doesn't seem to be sore the following day. Exercise also is important, even for older dogs, for maintaining muscle tone and keeping joints limber. However, overuse can aggravate the joints and accelerate degeneration.

Swimming can be an ideal exercise for dogs with arthritis because it allows movement of the joints with the support of the water to reduce the effects of gravity. Be sure your dog is comfortable in the water and supervise the exercise. Afterward, rinse the coat with warm water and clean the ears with special ear cleaning and drying solution to prevent ear infections.

Medical therapy using anti-inflammatory drugs

such as aspirin or even steroids is the most common approach to treatment of arthritis. Dosage of such medications is very different for humans, so it is important to consult a veterinarian before starting treatment. Side effects caused by incorrect doses of such drugs include vomiting, stomach irritation, bleeding ulcers, decreased ability of the blood to clot and kidney problems.

Some researchers believe that liquid food supplements with high concentrations of marine lipids (fish oils) and borage oil together can help control arthritis pain and inflammation in dogs. Vitamin E in the diet also can be important to help mobilize the joints.

Never give a pet any of your own medications, such as Tylenol, Advil or Motrin. These drugs can be extremely toxic to pets and never should be used unless under direct medical supervision. Aspirin and Tylenol can kill cats and never should be used in their treatment.

Surgery can be very beneficial in alleviating joint pain, increasing joint function and correcting instabilities for certain types of degenerative joint diseases. For example, it is now fairly common for dogs to have total hip replacements.

Autoimmune Disease

Q: My dog has a skin problem that our veterinarian calls pemphigus. My sister

**suffers from a disease called lupus. Is it
true that these conditions are related?**

A: The medical conditions that you mention are both forms of autoimmune disease. The body's immune system gets confused and starts attacking its own cells instead of fighting off bacteria and viruses.

Autoimmune diseases occur in both humans and animals. Lupus can involve many organ systems. Sometimes autoimmune diseases can be limited to specific organs, such as blood, joints and kidneys. The skin disease that has affected your dog, pemphigus, is an example of an organ-specific autoimmune disease, usually affecting only the skin.

In autoimmune skin diseases, the antibodies will attack so the skin cells lose the "glue" that holds them together. The result is skin blisters, crusts and ulcers that affect any skin but especially the face, ears, feet and foot pads.

Diagnosis of this form of autoimmune disease is made from skin biopsies and a special test called immunofluorescence that causes the abnormal cells to light up under laboratory examination. Other forms of autoimmune disease are diagnosed primarily by blood tests.

Some autoimmune diseases are aggravated and possibly even caused by sun exposure, especially on light skinned areas of a pet's nose. Waterproof sun block is a must for all pink or white skin that gets exposed to the sun.

Collies and Shetland sheepdogs can develop sores, especially on their faces, when they suffer from an inherited autoimmune disease called dermatomyositis.

"Dermato" refers to inflammation of the skin, and "myositis" is an inflammation of the muscles. Cells in both the skin and muscles are attacked and damaged or destroyed by other cells in the animal's own immune system.

Unfortunately, dermatomyositis cannot be effectively treated with steroids or other anti-inflammatory medications. Dogs that have mild skin lesions and little or no muscle weakness usually grow strong and develop into normal adults. Those animals with severe skin sores and strong evidence of muscle problems will not do well and may have to be euthanized.

Most other autoimmune diseases typically are treated with drugs which suppress the immune systems, such as cortisone, some anti-cancer medications and even injections of gold salts.

Although autoimmune diseases are not curable, many can be treated and controlled to increase your pet's comfort and quality of life.

Back Problems

Q: I have a dachshund who has problems with her back. She will seem to be OK for awhile, but then she will have a spell where she is in a lot of pain. What can be done?

A: Degenerative disc disease is the most common cause of chronic back problems in both dogs and humans.

Dogs with backs that are very long, compared to the length of their legs, are especially prone to experience back problems. Breeds that often suffer from disc disease include dachshunds, Pekinese, miniature poodles, cocker spaniels and beagles.

The back bones (vertebrae) are cushioned from each other by discs made of material that is the consistency of crab meat. When this disc material gets pushed out and puts pressure on the spinal cord or spinal nerves, it is called a slipped disc or a ruptured disc.

The result of a ruptured disc usually is soreness, pain and instability of the back. Other symptoms include weakness, lack of coordination, loss of feeling and inability to move. In extreme cases, complete paralysis, total collapse or loss of bladder functions can result.

Nerves of the spinal cord must be able to carry messages both to and from the animal's brain. The extruded disc material puts pressure on the nerves and interferes with nerve transmission.

Urgent medical care is required. Your veterinarian can judge the degree of injury to the nerves during the physical exam. X-rays probably will be necessary.

In many cases, restricted activity and appropriate

doses of aspirin or other anti-inflammatory medication can control the discomfort. However, if there is any loss of feeling in a foot or leg in addition to back pain when your pet moves, the spinal cord injury probably is severe and the chance for recovery is poor.

Surgery can relieve the pressure on the spinal cord if the damage is not extensive. A veterinary neurologist should be consulted when possible.

Bathing Your Pet

Q: My dogs always seem to have dandruff and dull coats. I either use baby shampoo or regular dish detergent on them, but I think it dries their skin. Any suggestions?

A: Dish detergents and shampoo intended for humans should never be used on dogs or cats. Your dogs have skin that is thinner and much more sensitive than human skin, and shampoos for humans have completely different pH levels.

There also is a big difference in the quality between various products that are available for bathing your pet, just as there are different qualities of human hair and skin care products. Poor quality ingredients, artificial coloring and cheap perfumes are used in many skin care products for pets. These products can be very drying, irritating and even cause allergic reactions, resulting in itching and various related skin problems.

Research indicates that high-quality hypoaller-genic shampoos, conditioners and food supplements achieve best results for skin and hair coat care when they are used in combination.

These products can be used either for dogs and cats that have dry skin like your pets, or in conjunc-tion with veterinary medical treatment of a variety of skin problems, including dermatitis related to al-lergies resulting from fleas, food and pollen.

The best shampoos are hypoallergenic, don't con-tain soap and are low lathering to gently clean your pet's hair coat while adding softness and body. The dandruff and scaling is removed, the skin is mois-turized and itching subsides.

Skin- and coat-conditioning sprays and afterbath rinses can help control itching by softening, mois-turizing and healing the damaged skin.

Pet food supplements should contain a combina-tion of marine lipids, borage oil, lecithin and essen-tial fatty acids, which are commonly destroyed by heat in the manufacture and storage of many pet foods. These nutrients cannot be produced by the body. Therefore, they should be added to the diet to boost the immune system, fight against allergic re-actions, and help control dandruff, dry hair coats and excessive shedding. Vitamins A and E also are important for healing.

Since dogs and cats have a wide variety of coat types, each pet should have an individual bathing schedule. Most dogs with normal skin and hair can be bathed just once a month.

Let your individual dogs tell you how often they should be bathed. After a bath using the hypoallergenic shampoo and conditioning afterbath, your pet's itching should be eliminated or significantly reduced. When the itching begins to return, whether in a week or a month, it's time for another bath. If the itching begins again within a day or two after a bath, there probably is an underlying medical problem that should be treated by a veterinarian. (See *Skin Care Products.*)

Behavior Problems

Q: My dog is very badly behaved. He barks constantly, rolls in terrible smelling things like dead birds and dog feces in the park, and never obeys me at all. What can I do?

A: Your dog needs to take classes from a professional animal trainer. He is just following his instincts without any discipline.

If hiring a private trainer or enrolling your dog in a class doesn't fit your budget, buy a book or video specifically on training your dog to behave.

For example, dogs cannot speak words, so they communicate with other sounds and actions. Dogs bark to communicate with you or other dogs. Sometimes the bark can be a greeting, a warning, or an expression of frustration or conflict. The excited bark when you return home or engage in play is very different from the bark, snarl and guttural growl to warn about the presence of a stranger. However, trained dogs will attack fearlessly without barking.

Every dog has a distinct personality. Some tend to be quiet and others very vocal. Dogs howl to bring the pack together to hunt or for protection. Pampered domestic dogs don't have the same need to howl, but the siren of a fire engine or ambulance can trigger some primitive urge that always seems to result in a neighborhood chorus of howling.

The basenji (African barkless dog) doesn't bark at all, and the wolf, a champion howler, just makes an unimpressive "wuff" sound instead of a bark.

The habit of rolling in excrement or the carcass of a dead animal is another instinctive action. Dogs often try to camouflage their scent for hunting prey. If your dog rolls in the decaying remains of a bird, he will smell more like the birds that he is chasing.

Another theory is that dogs just enjoy rolling in strong smelling substances—sort of a canine "perfume." Using a leash when you take your dog to the park may be necessary to prevent this type of behavior.

Bladder Stones

Q: My dog has bladder stones and might need an operation that I can't afford. Is there any alternative?

A: There are several different kinds of bladder stones. If your pet has the kind most commonly found in female dogs, her medical problem might be controlled simply by a change to a special prescription diet.

Bladder stones are formed of crystals in different shapes, materials, sizes and colors. More than 80 percent of the bladder stones found in female dogs are made of crystals called struvite, which look like prisms. These stones appear white on an X-ray.

A urinalysis can help to determine if your pet's bladder problem is a result of struvite stones. If so, a prescription diet (available through many veterinarians) can be used initially to dissolve crystals and stones.

Most dogs with struvite crystals have a bladder infection that also must be treated with antibiotics while the stones are being dissolved and for as long as four weeks afterward. Most symptoms disappear within a week, but the length of treatment varies with the size and number of stones.

After all of the bladder stones dissolve, another prescription diet can be used to prevent recurrence of the disease. This diet reduces the amount of magnesium, phosphorus and ammonium in the diet, and helps your pet maintain an appropriate level of acid in the urine.

Some bladder stones won't respond well to a prescription diet, and surgery becomes the only other option.

Bleeding Disorder

Q: My Doberman puppy recently got a nosebleed and sometimes her gums bleed, too. My vet wants to test to see if she has a bleeding disorder. What could cause that?

A: The most common bleeding disorder found in dogs is called von Willebrand's disease, and it is especially prevalent in Dobermans, Scottish terriers and Shelties.

The disease is caused by a defect in a protein substance called von Willebrand's factor, which is supposed to act like glue so that platelets can cause normal blood to clot if there is a cut or wound.

Dogs with von Willebrand's disease often bleed excessively from the mouth or nose, or have bloody urine. Because their blood doesn't clot normally, they bleed too long after surgery or any kind of trauma.

Von Willebrand's disease is inherited. If the dog has received the defective gene from both parents and produces no von Willebrand's factor, the bleeding tendency will be severe. If the disease is inherited from just one parent, the bleeding tendency can be greatly reduced because some von Willebrand's factor protein substance is present.

Doberman puppies sometimes can develop noticeable bleeding signs. The Scotties and shelties usually are about twelve to eighteen months old when the disease becomes noticeable.

Your veterinarian can diagnose von Willebrand's disease by using a special blood test, but there is no cure. Most dogs that have this condition will need supportive medical treatment for excessive bleeding from time to time. Puppies with von Willebrand's disease sometimes bleed badly when they start teething or if they traumatize their tails or ears by scratching or chewing themselves to satisfy an itch.

Dogs with this disease should be kept out of situations in which they might be bitten or scratched by other animals. Also, if possible, these dogs should not be left alone for long periods of time because they could bleed to death from fairly simple wounds if they don't receive prompt medical care.

Also, extreme care must be taken if a dog that suffers from von Willebrand's disease ever requires surgery.

Bloat

Q: I go jogging with my Great Dane every evening, but lately he seems uncomfortable after we run and sometimes belches. Could the exercise be causing a problem?

A: Air that your dog swallows during exercise just before or soon after eating can cause problems if it becomes trapped in the stomach and expands without being released.

The trapped air can result in a condition called gastric dilatation or "bloat," which happens most often in large breed dogs and is even more common in bigger animals like cows and horses.

Sometimes the stomach also will twist, causing further complications. These torsions are extremely dangerous and often can be fatal.

Bloat is a medical emergency. The first sign of the problem usually is a sudden distended, painful abdomen. The dog may be restless and try unsuccessfully to vomit.

As the stomach continues to expand, it cuts off the blood supply to internal organs, and the blood also is prevented from returning to the heart to get oxygen. The larger the stomach gets, the less space the lungs have to expand and fill with air. Breathing therefore becomes increasingly difficult. The dog might go into shock because of the lack of oxygen.

A veterinarian will give immediate medical treatment by passing a tube down the throat into the stomach in an attempt to relieve the pressure.

If the stomach is twisted, the tube usually will not pass all the way. In these cases, the stomach must be entered surgically through the abdomen. Treatment for shock includes fluids given through an intravenous catheter.

X-rays are taken to evaluate the position of the stomach and to help determine if it is actually twisted. Heart complications are fairly common, especially in the form of abnormal heart rates. An electrocardiogram (ECG) is used to monitor the heartbeat and rhythm. Often medication is needed to correct any abnormal rhythm.

After the dog is stabilized from shock, surgery can be performed. First the stomach is decompressed, allowing the trapped gases to escape. Then it can be untwisted and inspected for areas of tissue damage which should be surgically removed. The spleen also may have to be removed if it is severely damaged. Next, the stomach is surgically sutured into place to help prevent a recurrence.

To help prevent bloat in large dogs, feed several smaller meals instead of one large meal. Water should not be given with meals. Also, avoid giving your pet food or water just before or just after exercise.

Blocked Cat (FUS)

Q: My male cat is having a lot of trouble urinating. Sometimes he just strains and nothing happens. Is there something that I should do to help correct the problem?

A: Take your pet to a veterinarian *immediately*—this is a medical emergency! Feline urological syndrome (FUS) is an inflammation of the bladder and urethra that can slow or completely stop normal urination. The problem can be fatal if left untreated for twelve to forty-eight hours because of the buildup of toxic wastes in the urine.

About 10 percent of all cats that are brought to veterinary hospitals suffer from this life-threatening problem. Prompt treatment by a veterinarian usually results in complete recovery.

Symptoms of FUS are prolonged squatting and straining when urinating, blood in the urine, more frequent urination than normal, urinating in unusual places, and a swollen, hard bladder that is painful to the touch. Cats with this problem tend to lose their appetites, act sluggish and even begin vomiting.

FUS occurs when mineral crystals form in the urine and irritate the urinary tract lining. Eventually they can plug the urethra. Male cats are especially prone to having a plugged urethra and obstruction when the urine cannot flow out of the bladder.

Increased concentration of these crystals typically is caused by infrequent urination due to a litter box that is dirty or difficult to reach, reduced drinking because of lack of available water, and high levels of certain minerals and ash in the diet.

When your cat's urinary tract is blocked, the veterinarian will immediately empty the bladder. Then, the cat will receive a physical exam to determine the best treatment. Depending on the severity of the case, the veterinarian may recommend fluid therapy to relieve dehydration and re-balance the blood chemistry, removal of mineral crystals blocking the urine, insertion of a urinary catheter and hospitalization. Surgery to increase the size of the urethra sometimes is recommended.

Follow-up therapy almost always consists of pre-scribing a low-magnesium diet which allows pro-duction of a normal acid urine to prevent formation of crystals.

The FUS inflammation occurs as often in female cats as in male cats, but the males are more at risk because their anatomy makes complete obstruction of the urine flow more likely.

Boarding Your Pet

Q: I have three cats and a dog. What precautions should I take before boarding my pets this summer?

A: Be sure to tour the kennel facility where your pets will stay and satisfy yourself that it is clean, comfortable and well-managed. Also, try to get an idea of whether your pets will be loved and cared for or simply kept and fed.

All reputable kennels insist that your pets are cur-rent on their vaccinations. Dogs should be up-to-date on the distemper-parvo combination, rabies, bordetella and corona vaccinations.

Parvovirus, for many years the leading fatal dis-ease among dogs before a vaccine was developed, occasionally mutates and stages a comeback in vari-ous areas of the country. Every dog should have the DHLP-P vaccination each year. Puppies are particu-larly vulnerable to distemper and the parvovirus.

Bordetella, or "kennel cough," is a common upper-respiratory infection that is very contagious and easily picked up in a kennel situation if dogs aren't vaccinated. This disease can develop into pneumonia.

The coronavirus is sometimes described as a weaker version of the parvovirus. But it can be just as deadly, especially if a dog has other medical problems or comes down with parvo and corona viruses at the same time.

Your cats should be current on the feline distemper combination (FVR-CP), feline infectious peritonitus (FIP) and rabies vaccinations. In addition, all cats should be tested for the deadly feline leukemia virus (FeLV) and feline AIDS (FIV). Any cats with these diseases should be boarded in isolation from other cats. If your cats test negative for feline leukemia, the FeLV vaccinations must be current. There is no vaccination for feline AIDS.

Many dog and cat owners plan to take their pets to the veterinarian about four weeks before leaving on vacation for a complete physical exam and any necessary vaccinations. That way they can be more confident that their pets are in good health and have proper protection while they are away.

Bone in Throat

Q: My husband always gives our dog chicken bones, and sometimes they get stuck in her throat. Isn't that dangerous?

A: Sharp bones and a wide variety of other sharp objects, like wood, glass or plastic, can become stuck in the airway or tear the esophagus, the pathway that leads from the mouth to the stomach.

All dogs love to chew on bones, and some even like to swallow unusual items such as nylons, string, avocado pits, buttons, golf balls and rubber bands. You name it, and it probably has found its way into some dog's stomach. Many of these objects can be swallowed without causing the pet to choke, but some will become lodged in the esophagus and others are sharp enough to cause a tear in the wall of the esophagus.

Even after successfully passing through the esophagus and the stomach, some objects still can cause problems. String and nylons, for example, can become entwined inside a pet's stomach or intestines, causing dangerous blockage.

Although dogs in the wild have plenty of bones to chew, domestic dogs generally are better off without them because of the potential danger. The exception is a large, uncooked knuckle bone that doesn't splinter. Chicken bones can be especially dangerous because they are so small and sharp. For most dogs, a chew toy can be a very satisfactory replacement for a bone.

Perforation of the esophagus can be a difficult condition to diagnose. The most common approach is for your veterinarian to use X-rays and a special dye to see if there are any leaks in the wall of the esophagus. There also may be signs of abnormal air trapped in the pet's chest.

Surgery to close such a perforation of the esophagus can be both difficult and risky.

Keeping your pet's environment free of potentially dangerous foreign objects and providing a safe chew toy is the best way to prevent choking and perforation of the esophagus.

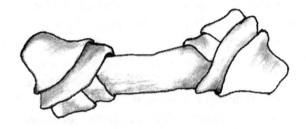

Breast Cancer

Q: My female poodle has several hard little lumps near one of her nipples. Do you think she could have breast cancer?

A: Female dogs can develop breast cancer, just like humans, especially as they start getting older. The incidence of breast cancer is dramatically reduced if your dog is spayed before her third heat cycle, usually between six and twelve months of age.

Breast cancer is the second most common malignancy seen in dogs. Only skin cancer is more widespread.

Any lumps anywhere on your pet's body should

be checked immediately by a veterinarian because the key to curing cancer is early diagnosis and treatment.

Your veterinarian will be able to determine if the lumps that you describe are dangerous malignant tumors or harmless benign tumors or cysts.

Breast cancer lumps usually are firm, dense and often near the nipple. Cancer masses can be movable or fixed underneath the skin and vary greatly in size. It may grow significantly and become open and sore within a few weeks. Other symptoms might include depression and weakness, fever, pale gums, decreased appetite or weight loss.

Your veterinarian may be able to feel masses in other breast tissue, indicating the spread of the main cancer mass. Small amounts of a brown, watery discharge may be squeezed from nipples of the involved glands. When studied under a microscope, this fluid may show cancer cells.

If breast cancer is suspected, your veterinarian will recommend a biopsy, blood work and X rays to determine if the mass is malignant and has spread to other parts of the body.

If there is no evidence of spread to the lungs, a partial or total mastectomy can be performed to remove the tumor and varying amounts of surrounding breast tissue.

Since hormones often affect the growth of the cancer, an ovariohysterectomy (spay) usually is recommended.

In addition, a vaccine sometimes is used to stimulate the animal's immune system to reduce the size of the cancer before surgery. Chemotherapy also may be recommended.

Early diagnosis and treatment of cancerous tumors can prolong a pet's life. Unfortunately, malignant tumors can grow rapidly and spread to other parts of the body.

Remember, if a female dog is spayed before one year of age, the risk of breast cancer is reduced dramatically.

Breeding Dogs

Q: I'm planning to breed my Labrador before I have her spayed. She is almost a year old and seems to be interested in males. How will I know exactly when to breed her?

A: Female dogs can come into heat, or the estrus cycle, as early as six months of age and as late as one year or more, depending on the breed.

When your dog starts her period, it is normal to notice a bloody vaginal discharge. Often dogs will tend to lick this area a lot. The bleeding phase is called proestrus—meaning before estrus. Proestrus usually will last ten to twelve days.

Estrus is the actual short period of time during which female dogs will mate. These are called the days of standing heat.

Prime days to breed usually are the tenth and

twelfth days after the proestrus bleeding starts or the first, third and fifth days of standing heat. When the vaginal discharge becomes a pale pink color rather than red blood, and the area around your pet's vagina becomes less swollen, she will be ready.

A veterinarian can study a vaginal smear under the microscope to detect changes in the cell structure as a female dog gets closer to the breeding time. Usually the smears are taken at intervals of one or two days. Also, the hormone levels can be measured to help determine breeding time. An experienced stud dog usually knows exactly when to mate with the female.

Be very certain about your decision to breed your pet. Both parent dogs should have complete physical exams and be healthy. Avoid breeding if either dog has such hereditary diseases as hip displasia, hypothyroidism, mange, certain eye problems, allergies or medical disorders that could be passed on to the puppies.

Also, make sure your dog is on a high-quality pet food recommended by your veterinarian. Make sure, too, that her diet is altered to compensate for specific nutritional needs during pregnancy and while she is nursing her puppies.

Cancer

Q. Three of my pets have died of cancer in the last two years. I'm worried that something in the environment might be causing this. How common is cancer in pets?

A: Dogs and cats get cancer just like humans do—and for most of the same reasons.

Cancer researchers are quite certain about three things: Cancer is influenced by genetic programming, so the tendency to get cancer can be hereditary; cancer can be influenced by various elements in the environment, including secondary cigarette smoke, radiation, radon gas, diet and toxic chemicals; and cancer takes advantage of weak immune systems, which in cats can be caused by such diseases as the feline leukemia virus (FeLV) or feline AIDS (FIV).

Cancers can affect any organ system. Primary cancers originate in one organ and then can spread or metastasize from one site to other organ systems by the blood or lymph systems.

Skin cancers are the most common type of tumors. Squamous cell carcinoma and basal cell tumors often are caused by excessive sun exposure, especially in white and pink-skinned dogs and cats. The cancers most often appear on the ears or noses, around the eyes and on sun-bathed tummies. Help your pet avoid the sun. Use waterproof No. 15 SPF sunblock on the exposed areas of your pet's skin.

Black dogs are susceptible to melanomas, which are cancers of the cells that produce pigment. Melanocytes can grow out of control in the mouth and skin causing a black mass or swelling. They are highly malignant.

Mast cell tumors occur commonly in the skin of older dogs, especially boxers and Boston terriers. If the mast cell spreads to the bone marrow and spleen, it is very serious.

The second most common type of cancer is mammary gland cancer in female dogs and cats. Breast cancers usually occur in older unspayed females. Spaying your female before her third heat cycle reduces the chance of breast cancer to almost zero. A mass or swelling may be the only sign of a tumor.

Blood cancers are the next most common forms of cancer. Leukemia is a cancer of the blood and bone marrow. It affects any of the white blood cells and in cats is caused by the feline leukemia virus (FeLV).

Bone tumors are more often seen in large or giant breed dogs.

Cancer of the lymph nodes is called lymphosarcoma. Lung cancer in pets can be caused by secondary cigarette smoke, just like in humans. Dogs with longer noses are less likely to develop lung cancer but more likely to develop nasal cancer, because the nose acts like a filtration system.

Male dogs sometimes develop cancer in a retained testicle. Females can suffer from ovarian cancer.

Tumors that develop around the eye tend to be

benign and grow slowly. However, squamous cell carcinomas may involve the skin around the eye and can be fatal.

There are several ways to help protect your pet from getting cancer:

• Have your pet spayed or neutered as soon as possible.

• Keep your pet away from secondary tobacco smoke and check your home for radon gas.

• Use waterproof sunblock on skin areas that are unprotected by the hair coat and exposed to the sun.

• Feed your pet a high-quality, premium food.

• Give your pet natural vitamin supplements formulated for a healthier, longer life. Whenever possible, avoid feeding your pet sugars, corn syrup, artificial colorings, flavorings and preservatives.

• Check your pet for lumps or masses under the skin and watch for such symptoms as weight loss, vomiting, diarrhea, behavior changes, increased or decreased water consumption or appetite, and unexplained bleeding.

• Annual physical exams by your veterinarian are very important, and senior pets should have checkups every six months.

Cancer treatments depend on the type of tumor and the stage that it has reached when diagnosed. Early diagnosis is always very important for successful treatment. Surgical removal of the tumor is the preferred treatment. However, if the tumor is diffuse or has spread, radiation and chemotherapy often are used.

Cataracts

Q: My ten-year-old dog's eyes have started looking cloudy, and I don't think she sees as well as she used to. Could she be getting cataracts?

A: All dogs over the age of about eight years develop a hazy appearance to the lenses of their eyes. This normal change is called sclerosis, and your pet's vision will not be affected. Sclerosis results when the lens adds onion-like layers and becomes more dense as the dog ages.

Cataracts, on the other hand, are the clouding of the normally clear lens of the eye which keeps light from passing through. Cataracts can be small or completely cover the lens, and vision may be lost in varying degrees.

Dogs can be born with cataracts or develop them as puppies or adults. Cataracts either can be inherited or caused by lack of proper nutrition, diseases such as diabetes or even drugs such as cortisone.

Dogs with diabetes develop cataracts because the high buildup of sugar causes a chemical reaction which eventually clouds lens tissue in the eye.

Some cataracts develop quite rapidly, while others grow very, very slowly. Regular examinations by a veterinarian are important to keep track of the rate of cataract development.

Cataract surgery is more difficult in dogs than humans because the lens in the eye of a dog is much larger and very sensitive. As a result, it can become inflamed, resulting in scarring and even blindness.

Surgery is not recommended to remove small cataracts. Usually surgery is performed only on dogs with severely affected vision or blindness in both eyes.

It is critical to consult a veterinary ophthalmologist to determine if the retina and optic nerve are functioning properly.

Cat Scratch Fever

Q: I was scratched by a stray cat in the neighborhood and ended up getting sick. Can you explain why this would happen?

A: Your physician is the best person to answer this question in your specific case, but some people get a rare disease commonly called "cat scratch fever" after being clawed or bitten by a cat.

Cat scratch fever is caused by a bacteria transmitted from the cat to the human, and results in swollen lymph nodes in the area of the wound. The disease usually just goes away by itself, although some people are affected for several months.

The cat that transmits cat scratch fever usually is a healthy, young animal. In extreme cases, people may develop a fever, sore throat and headache. A skin pimple or red, raised papule may form three to ten days after the contact with the cat. Swollen lymph nodes usually last for several weeks.

Your physician can diagnose cat scratch fever based on the medical history, a skin test or sometimes a biopsy.

There are more than fifty million pet cats in the United States, and only a small number of people are diagnosed as having cat scratch fever each year.

Cats That Hunt

Q: My cat is a great hunter, but he constantly drags home disgusting dead creatures—mice, lizards and birds—and leaves them on my porch. Is that normal?

A: Throughout history, cats have been known for their hunting skills. During the 11th Century when the dreaded Black Plague swept Europe, cats were especially in demand because they were so effective in hunting the rats that carried the fleas that spread the disease.

Cats ambush their prey. Usually the hunter slinks along with tail twitching until the victim is within striking range. Then the cat pounces and holds its prey down with the front paws to make the kill. The spinal cord is severed, which paralyzes the victim.

Hunting techniques are taught to kittens by the mother cat and are practiced during play. If a kitten fails to catch the prey, the mother cat usually will capture the mouse or other victim herself and bring it to the kitten.

Cats are able to hunt at night because of a surface called the tapetum on the back of the eye that allows light to be reflected. They need only a fraction of the light required by a human to see, but cats have blurred vision and are almost color blind. However, they have tremendous peripheral vision and the ability to notice even the slightest movement.

Siamese cats often have crossed eyes and abnormal nerve connections to the center of the brain, which results in difficulty locating objects.

Cats rely on their whiskers to help them find prey at night, using them to measure distances from an object or to detect wind and air currents. The top two rows of whiskers move independently of the bottom two rows on a cat's face. When the cat is walking, the whiskers are thrust forward and out to the sides. During a greeting, defense or sniff, they are folded back along the side of the head.

Your talented hunter is just following his instincts and then trying to get some attention from you for his accomplishments.

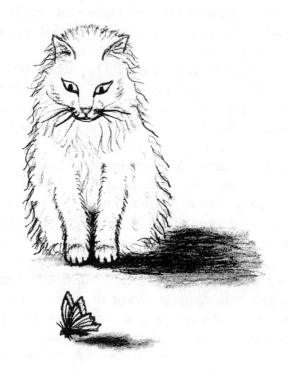

Cherry Eye

**Q: I have a Lhasa apso puppy that suddenly
has developed a bright red lump in the corner
of one eye. She doesn't seem bothered by it.
Should I be worried?**

A: Based on your description, the puppy might
have a condition called cherry eye which usually is
seen in young, small breed dogs.

The third eyelid, which is located at the inside

corner of each eye, helps to keep the eye clean and moist. The red lump that you see is actually the gland of the third eyelid that has become exposed. When the fibers that attach the gland are weakened or defective, it can cause the red, swollen, "cherry eye" appearance.

This condition looks unsightly and can be very uncomfortable for your pet. In some cases, cherry eye can cause severe irritation to the surface of the eye and eventually might result in loss of vision.

Cherry eye can be repaired with surgery. The veterinary surgeon should be careful not to remove any tear-producing tissue so the eye will remain moist and healthy.

Coronavirus

Q: What exactly is the coronavirus? Is it as deadly as the parvovirus?

A: Like the notorious parvovirus, the coronavirus can cause diarrhea, vomiting and dehydration in dogs - and it can be just as deadly.

The coronavirus is extremely contagious and spreads rapidly among exposed dogs. It is not uncommon for all unvaccinated dogs in a kennel or a household to come down with the virus within a day or two after one of them is exposed. The first symptoms are depression, lack of appetite and vomiting. Diarrhea usually follows a day or two later.

Coronavirus, like parvovirus, is most severe in puppies.

Because both coronavirus and parvovirus have many of the same symptoms, it is difficult to distinguish between them without a lab test. Dogs can come down with both diseases at once, which sharply reduces their chances for recovery.

Because puppies are so susceptible to both diseases, they should get their first vaccinations at eight weeks of age. Booster vaccinations also are given at three week intervals until the puppy is at least sixteen weeks old, and then annually. Adult dogs should receive one vaccination and then a booster in three to four weeks. Female dogs should get a booster vaccination three weeks before breeding.

Parvo is routinely included with the distemper combination vaccination, often called the 5-in-1 vaccination or DHLP-P. But be sure to ask your veterinarian specifically to give the coronavirus vaccination, too, because it may not be included in the combination vaccination.

Crossed-eyes

Q: I'm planning to get a little two-month-old Siamese kitten, but I think she might not be purebred because her eyes aren't crossed. Don't all Siamese cats have crossed eyes?

A: Siamese and Himalayan cats have a gene that

causes abnormal nerve connections in the visual pathways between their eyes and their brains. This causes part of their visual field to be inverted - just the opposite of normal. In addition, all Siamese cats lack binocular vision, the ability to form one picture from two eyes. The result is their typical cross-eyed appearance.

Siamese cats compensate for this misinformation by "rewiring" their brains. This condition reduces their visual precision, so they don't see quite as well as other cats.

Siamese cats typically develop their cross-eyed look during the third month of life, as their brains try to create a complete visual field by changing the position of the eyes. The muscles supporting the eyes become accustomed to this position and the cross-eyed look becomes permanent.

The gene that causes the crossed eyes also is responsible for the beautiful coat color combinations in the Siamese and Himalayan breeds. The color variations are caused by pigment production that changes with temperature. More pigment is produced in areas where there is greater heat loss, such as the legs and tail.

Because Siamese cats are deficient in pigment production, they lack pigment on the retinas at the back of their eyes, a condition which also affects their eyesight.

Declawing Cats

Q: Our indoor cats are destroying the furniture, and my husband insists that we either get them declawed or put them to sleep. Isn't it cruel to have cats declawed?

A: Declawing is a very safe surgical procedure that is probably about as uncomfortable for cats as many common elective cosmetic surgeries are for humans. And if the alternative is getting rid of your cats - or your husband - you should consider the option of having your indoor cats declawed.

Cats have a natural instinct to sharpen their claws. Often a carpet-covered scratching post will satisfy them, and regular toenail trims will minimize damage to your furniture and curtains. Cats that are allowed to go outdoors at any time should not be declawed because their claws are critical for escaping from and defending themselves against other cats, dogs and wild animals in your neighborhood.

Indoor cats, however, have no real need for their claws. Declawing an indoor cat can greatly improve the quality of your life by saving your furniture and drapes, and, as a result, improve the quality of your cat's life.

Each year, many cats are abused physically or even put to sleep just because they followed their natural instincts to sharpen their claws and accidentally ruined expensive pieces of furniture.

When your cat is declawed, your veterinarian will

use a general anesthetic, making the surgery pain-less. The paws will be sore for a few days and usu-ally are kept bandaged to help prevent bleeding and infection. Some veterinarians prefer to keep the cats hospitalized during this time to minimize activities that might cause the bandages to come off.

Once your declawed cats are home, it is impor-tant to keep their feet clean. They should not be al-lowed outside, and your veterinarian may want you to use shredded white paper rather than litter or sand for several days to prevent particles from getting into the surgical site and causing infection.

The best time to declaw cats is while they are be-ing spayed or neutered - at about six to eight months. This allows two surgical procedures to be done un-der one anesthetic, which is safer for the cat and more economical for you.

Dental Problems

Q: One of my dogs has lots of dental problems, including tartar, loose teeth and bad breath. My other dog has perfect teeth. What could cause the difference?

A: Dogs with different genetic histories can have very different medical and dental problems, even if they live in the same environment and eat the same food. Some dogs have teeth that need regular atten-tion - brushing, chew toys, special diets and dentistries twice a year. Other dogs have strong, healthy teeth all of their lives.

However, an annual dental examination is very important for all dogs. Excessive tartar on the teeth, especially at the gum line, can result in irritation, infection and receding gums. This can lead to serious infections and diseases of the gums and teeth, as well as digestion and nutritional problems, which cause bad breath. When dental problems are ignored and left untreated, bacteria can build up in your dog's mouth and lead to other infections in the body - including in the heart.

Other common symptoms of tooth and gum disease include decreased appetite, sneezing, and a reluctance to eat hard food. During an examination, your veterinarian may find red, sore, or receded gums; loose, infected teeth; yellow-brown tartar on the teeth; and even infected sinuses.

Pets with excessive tartar or infected teeth or gums are due for dentistries. A general anesthesia is required to thoroughly clean your pet's teeth. Any loose, infected teeth are pulled and the infected areas are treated. After being cleaned, the healthy teeth are polished. Antibiotics often are necessary to fight infection and may be started a few days before the dentistry to help protect against infection spreading in the bloodstream.

Many pet owners elect to have a dentistry done when their pet is already under anesthesia for a spay or neuter surgery. A pre-anesthetic blood test always is recommended to help prevent unexpected complications.

In addition to dentistries, brushing your pet's teeth can be helpful in preventing dental disease. Pet stores and veterinary clinics carry toothbrushes and toothpastes specifically designed for dogs.

If you find that it is impractical to brush your pet's teeth, you should provide a diet that includes dry kibble to help reduce tartar buildup. Letting your dog have rawhide chew toys can help keep teeth healthy, but care should be taken not to permit your pet to chew on anything that might splinter and get stuck in the throat.

Periodically rubbing your pet's gums with a soft washcloth or gauze soaked in hydrogen peroxide helps clean away bacteria and other debris.

Diabetes

Q: I have an eight-year-old cat that has always been chubby. Recently she started drinking lots of water and eating more food than ever - yet she is losing weight. Why?

A: There are various medical problems which can cause dogs and cats to lose weight while increasing their intake of food and water. One of the most common, especially among older cats that have a weight problem, is diabetes mellitus. Diabetes is an inability to produce or use insulin properly.

Low insulin levels result in an increase in the cat's blood sugar. When the blood sugar levels get too high, the sugar spills over into the urine. The body essentially begins starving for energy when the sugar is lost in the urine.

If left untreated, diabetes can be fatal. The early symptoms include weight loss, weakness, excessive hunger and thirst, and excessive urination. Eventually, acids can build up in the blood, which may result in vomiting, coma and death.

Your veterinarian can test for diabetes with a blood panel and a urinalysis. Diabetes in cats and dogs is controlled the same way as in humans - usually with a special diet and insulin injections given each day at home.

Pets with diabetes must have a very consistent diet, with exactly the same kinds and amounts of food at each meal. Your veterinarian can provide a prescription diet designed specifically for pets with diabetes.

Your veterinarian also will show you how to give insulin to your cat each day. Learning to inject insulin under your cat's skin is not difficult after a little practice. In addition, you will need to test your cat's urine daily to determine the proper doses of insulin. Always keep some sugar syrup available to rub on your pet's gums if her blood sugar ever unexpectedly drops too low, causing convulsions.

Your cat's blood sugar levels will be tested periodically in the veterinary hospital to make sure she is stabilized and on a maintenance level of insulin.

If your pet's insulin level is kept under control, she can live a fairly normal life. However, cats with diabetes are prone to have suppressed immune systems, making them more susceptible to infections, cataracts and other medical problems.

Diabetes usually occurs in animals older than six years of age. Spaying or neutering often is recommended for pets with diabetes because hormones can affect the level of insulin in their bodies.

Diarrhea

Q: My little dog is very high-strung and gets nervous easily. She seems healthy, but sometimes gets diarrhea when she is stressed. Should I change her diet?

A: Nervous pets, just like nervous people, sometimes get upset stomachs or develop other medical problems related to the digestion of their food. Recurring diarrhea is a symptom that should be checked by your veterinarian.

One of the most common causes of occasional diarrhea is colitis, an inflammation of the colon, located in the lower part of the digestive tract. Pet owners usually observe their pets straining to have a bowel movement and notice increased frequency of loose stools or diarrhea with blood and mucous.

In addition to prescription medication, a diet high in fiber can be very beneficial for dogs and cats with colitis. The fiber allows the intestine to process and absorb food much better and reduces irritation from toxins. The pet's stool becomes more regular, drier and softer.

Dietary fiber is a general term for different forms of plant material that don't digest well in the small intestine. Instead, the fiber passes on through the digestive tract, improving water absorption and helping to keep elimination regular. Main sources of fiber include vegetables, wheat, oats and other grains, fruit and legumes.

Research indicates that the best diet for your pet should include complex carbohydrates and be low in fat, in addition to plenty of fiber. This diet not only is beneficial in the treatment of colitis, but is strongly recommended if your pet has diabetes or heart disease. Fiber also can prevent colon cancer.

The best way to provide this fiber to your cat and dog is in a high-quality, nutritionally balanced pet food. Since there are many commercial pet foods on the market that don't meet these standards, be sure to ask your veterinarian for a recommendation about which diet to use for your particular pet. Special prescription diets are available.

Your veterinarian also will want to test for intestinal parasites, a common cause of diarrhea.

Ear Problems

Q: My bassett hound is constantly scratching at her ears. They always smell awful, and she gets terrible infections. What can I do to prevent this?

A: Dogs, such as bassett hounds, with large, drooping ears or those with lots of hair in the ear canal often suffer with ear infections and inflammation even more than other breeds.

The ear canal of a dog lends itself to all kinds of medical problems because it makes a sharp right angle not far below the external opening. This bend in the canal traps wax, fluids and foreign bodies, all of which promote the growth of bacteria and yeast. As a result, ear infections are common.

Other typical causes of ear problems include allergies, mites and ticks.

The signs of ear problems can come on suddenly or be long-standing. The inside of your pet's ear might look red, swollen and ulcerated. There might be a bad odor and a waxy or even pus-like discharge. Since ear infections are painful, and allergies cause severe itching, the animal often will paw or scratch at the ears, shake its head, or cry if you touch around the ears.

Some animals even scratch so much that they cause bleeding between the inside and outside layers of the skin, resulting in swelling called a hematoma, which requires surgical treatment. It is very important to determine the actual cause of the ear problem. Your veterinarian will take a sample of the discharge from the ears with a swab to check under the microscope to determine if there are bacteria, yeast or mites. It may be necessary to submit the sample for a culture and sensitivity test to determine the most effective drug.

An otoscopic examination of the ear allows a close look at the canal and ear drum. Depending on your pet's disposition, she may need to be tranquilized or anesthetized for this exam or for cleaning, flushing or removing foreign bodies or ticks.

Cleaning and flushing infected ears initially should be done at a veterinary clinic and then followed up at home. Many cases require several weeks of treatment. The best possible results are obtained by following a regular step-by-step procedure to clean, dry and medicate the infected ears with products prescribed by the veterinarian. Oral antibiotics also may be needed.

In some long-standing cases, surgical exposure of the ear canal may be needed to allow drainage.

To prevent ear problems, keep the ears clean and dry, and treat the underlying causes. If ear infections are not treated, they can lead to severe ear problems with the loss of balance and deafness.

Emergencies

Q: When my pets get sick, how do I know if I should take them to a veterinarian immediately or just take care of them at home?

A: Most medical problems are not emergencies, but it is better to be cautiously safe than sorry. Therefore, it is important for you to be able to recognize potentially life-threatening situations.

The following symptoms are danger signals that should get prompt medical attention:

- Balance problems or lack of coordination.
- Bleeding from any part of the body, including blood in the urine and feces.
- Bloated abdomen.
- Breathing difficulty.
- Burns of any kind.
- Coughing or sneezing excessively.
- Choking, gagging or swallowing a foreign body.
- Collapse or unusual weakness.
- Dental problems, including mouth odor, loose teeth, gums that are purplish or pale white.
- Depression or hiding.
- Diarrhea that lasts more than twenty-four hours.
- Ear problems, including discharge, odor, soreness, head tilt, head shaking or foreign bodies.
- Eye injuries or irritations of any kind. Clouding of the eyes.
- Fever. Normal for a dog or cat is 101° to 102°.
- Fractures or possible fractures.

- Growths, lumps or masses under the skin.
- Paralysis or sudden inability to move legs.
- Panting excessively for an extended period.
- Pain expressed by crying, unusual growling, yelping, trembling or sensitivity to touch.
- Poisoning from ingested plants, medications, household pesticides or other toxic substances.
- Seizures, usually characterized by sudden weak ness, shaking and collapse.
- Shock, including loss of consciousness.
- Skin problems, including itching, scratching, licking, black or red skin, infected "hot spots," excessive shedding or hair loss.
- Swelling of abdomen, face, joint, leg or mouth.
- Trauma. For example, being hit by a car, falling or being attacked by another animal.
- Urination problems, including severe straining or complete inability to urinate, blood in the urine, excessive urination or urination in inap propriate places.
- Vaginal discharge with unusual blood or pus.
- Vomiting that is violent and continuous, or that lasts off and on for more than twenty-four hours.
- Water consumption that is significantly increased or decreased.
- Significant increase or decrease in weight.

Epilepsy

Q: My two-year-old poodle has had two episodes where she shakes violently and then collapses. Could she have epilepsy?

A: Poodles are more prone than most other breeds to suffer from epileptic seizures, which can result in the symptoms that you describe.

An epileptic seizure is a recurring abnormal electrical pattern in the brain that can cause a variety of symptoms, including muscle spasms, shaking or collapse.

Sometimes head injuries or the effects of medical problems such as liver or kidney disease or even distemper can result in epilepsy, although often the cause is unknown. Inheritance definitely plays a role in many cases. Epileptic dogs should never be used for breeding purposes.

There are three stages of an epileptic seizure. In the aura stage, or preseizure, the animal can sense the onset and may act restless or show abnormal behavior such as whining, hiding or pacing. This stage may occur minutes or days before the seizure.

The second stage, an actual seizure, usually lasts only a few minutes. In addition to shaking, your pet may run in circles, experience rhythmic muscle contractions or facial twitching, salivate, urinate, defecate, vomit, paddle wildly with the legs or completely collapse.

The third stage, or recovery, can last for several

hours or several days. Some animals seem disoriented or uncoordinated, and occasionally temporary blindness occurs. Other animals show virtually no symptoms except fatigue during the recovery stage.

Your veterinarian should give your pet a complete physical examination and probably will recommend blood tests and X rays to determine if there is a specific cause of the seizures other than a hereditary epilepsy. If an infection or tumor is not discovered, medication can be given to prevent or control abnormal electrical patterns in the brain.

Epileptic seizures often become more frequent and violent if they are not treated, so it is important to seek medical help for your pet as soon as possible. Sometimes epileptic episodes can be so severe that anti-seizure medication must be injected directly into a vein to avoid a coma, irreversible brain damage or even death.

When your pet has a seizure, remain calm and avoid getting bitten. Do not interfere other than removing any sharp objects from the area that might cause injury to your pet. If the seizure lasts for more than five minutes, call your veterinarian for emergency help.

Euthanasia

Q: My dear old dog is so feeble that she can't get up the stairs anymore, and she has lost her bladder control. I'm afraid that she is suffering. Should I have her put to sleep?

A: Whether or not to euthanize a beloved pet is often one of the most difficult decisions that you will ever have to face. The moment may come when an animal that has been your loyal companion, your trusting friend and a beloved member of your family for many years will look into your eyes and communicate unbearable pain and helplessness. When a pet is suffering that way and there is no hope of a comfortable life in the future, the euthanasia option can be a real blessing.

Dogs and cats are put to sleep for a variety of reasons. The most common cause, of course, is failing health. Diseases such as cancers or failure of the liver, kidneys or heart are progressive, resulting in poor quality of life, suffering and eventually death. Euthanasia is a way to prevent the suffering.

However, some people insist on euthanasia as the solution for pets that have behavior problems or because the owners can no longer keep them. Although there are no legal or professional criteria for precisely when euthanasia is appropriate for a pet, most veterinarians abide by their own convictions—sometimes refusing to euthanize dogs or cats unless there is a compelling medical reason.

When your pet is no longer able to live a happy, comfortable life, you and your veterinarian should discuss the euthanasia option. The procedure is quite literally "putting your pet to sleep."

A syringe is filled with a liquid anesthetic which is then injected into the pet's vein. The anesthetic not only gently puts the animal to sleep but also causes all of the vital organs to stop functioning— without any pain or suffering.

Euthanasia can be a traumatic emotional process for the pet owner. Some feel that it is important for them to be present during the injection, but for others the experience is too disturbing. Even though the animals don't feel any pain, they may moan, lose bladder control or even experience some muscle twitching. These are normal body reactions and do not indicate any suffering.

In many cases, owners are more easily able to overcome their feelings of grief and sadness at the loss of a beloved pet by providing a home for another similar animal that might otherwise be destroyed.

Fat Cat

Q: One of my cats is very fat. She weighs about twenty pounds and keeps on gaining. What kind of diet can you recommend?

A: Several questions need to be answered before

recommending a specific diet. First, it is important to determine why your cat is gaining weight.

Have you been overfeeding her or giving her table scraps and other treats? Is she raiding trash cans or scavenging the food dishes of your other pets? Do the neighbors feed her or does she hunt mice or birds for extra food? Is she getting older, with a correspondingly slower metabolism, but still being fed the same as when she was young?

You also should be aware that some medical problems, including brain disorders, hormone imbalances and psychological distress, can result in obesity.

Overweight pets are more prone to heart and lung disease, diabetes, pancreatitis (inflammation of the pancreas) and arthritis. They also are at much higher risk during surgery than animals of normal weight, and recovery often is slower.

After weighing your cat accurately, your veterinarian will discuss with you how many pounds she should lose and whether a special reducing diet is recommended. Many pet food companies now produce lower calorie foods for pets with weight problems. Reducing diet foods contain higher dietary fiber to help your cat feel full. They also have reduced fat content.

Another way to slim your cat down is to decrease the amount of regular food by about 20 percent and eliminate all table food and treats. Since your cat at first may complain bitterly, you can replace some of the volume of food with cooked vegetables like squash and carrots that are blended and mixed with the regular food. A teaspoon of tuna packed in water, along with the vegetables and the reduced amount of regular cat food, can be a favorite diet meal. Surprisingly, most cats like the vegetables.

Weigh your cat each week. A conscientious diet can result in a much happier, healthier and more attractive pet.

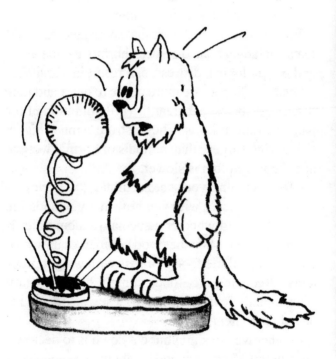

Feline AIDS

Q: I read that AIDS in cats is spreading. Is that disease the same as AIDS in humans? Can cats give AIDS to people?

A: Feline AIDS is extremely contagious to other cats—but not to other species such as humans, dogs or birds.

Recent studies show that about 3 percent of all healthy cats and up to 15 percent of chronically ill cats now have the feline AIDS virus (FIV). All cat owners should have their pets tested for this disease before it becomes an epidemic like the related feline leukemia virus (FeLV).

The FIV disease in cats is much like AIDS in humans, causing a deficiency in the immune system and making the cat susceptible to a wide variety of life-threatening medical problems.

The feline AIDS virus invades individual cells in the cat's body and then uses the genetic material of the cells to produce more viruses. Once a cell has been infected with the virus, it will remain infected for the rest of the cat's life. Therefore, once a cat tests positive for feline AIDS, no matter how much the immune system fights the disease, the body can never get rid of the virus.

Feline AIDS can result in poor appetite, weight loss, a poor coat, generally unhealthy appearance, diarrhea, and chronic infections of the gums, mouth, skin, sinuses and lungs. Some cats will develop anemia or abnormal neurological signs such as seizures.

Researchers know the virus is in saliva and blood, but they are still learning how it is transmitted. Older male cats spending the majority of time outdoors have been at greatest risk.

Unlike AIDS in humans, sexual contact doesn't seem to spread the feline version of the disease. Bite wounds seem to be a major means of infection, and infected mother cats can transmit the virus to their kittens. However, sharing food dishes and mutual grooming doesn't seem to be a problem.

The best way to prevent the spread of this deadly disease is to have your cat tested for feline AIDS, as well as the feline leukemia virus (FeLV). If your pet is a carrier, it should not be allowed to expose other cats. Spaying or neutering your pet will help reduce territorial fighting and also prevent the birth of infected kittens.

Feline Infectious Anemia

Q: My three-year-old cat looks yellow around his eyes and seems to feel sick. My vet says he has blood parasites. Can you explain?

A: Certain parasites can live in the bloodstreams of animals and destroy the red blood cells. It is thought that these parasites can be transmitted to your pet by insects that bite or suck blood.

One such parasite is hemobartonella, which causes a disease in cats called feline infectious anemia. Your veterinarian can identify this parasite by using a microscope to study a blood sample smear.

The hemobartonella parasite attaches to the edge of the red blood cells, which results in a severe anemia, pale to yellow mucous membranes and an enlarged spleen. These changes typically make the pet depressed, weak and feverish.

Hemobartonella most commonly affects young male cats like your pet. It is responsible for about 10 percent of all feline anemia cases.

Infected cats must be treated or the disease can be fatal. Treatment usually includes oral antibiotics, steroids and supportive care. Blood transfusions may be necessary for some animals.

Just like malaria in people, the hemobartonella parasite remains in the bloodstream of the carrier animal even after the pet recovers from anemia.

Relapses of hemobartonella can occur, especially if the cat is stressed, but otherwise there are no symptoms to indicate that the pet is a carrier of the parasite. Hemobartonella cannot be transferred to humans.

All cats with the hemobartonella parasite should be tested for the feline leukemia virus (FeLV). Sometimes cats can pass on both infections to their newborn kittens.

Feline Leukemia Virus (FeLV)

Q: I have five cats and it is very expensive to get vaccinations for all of them. How important are feline leukemia boosters?

A: The spread of feline leukemia virus (FeLV) is a true epidemic—and this deadly disease has become one of the main killers of cats throughout the world.

FeLV is highly contagious and easily can be transmitted from one cat to another in saliva, urine and feces. There is no known cure.

The feline leukemia virus causes an acquired immune deficiency, resulting in the destruction of the animal's immune system. This leaves the cat susceptible to a wide variety of cancers, infections and diseases.

A simple blood test can determine if your cat carries the feline leukemia virus. If the test is positive, your cat has been exposed to the virus and should be isolated from all other cats. However, this doesn't necessarily mean that your cat will become ill and die. Some cats are able to fight off the virus and become immune to it. Other cats that remain chronically infected with the virus usually die from infectious diseases not directly related to the virus because of weakened immune systems.

Vaccinations against FeLV consist of a series of three initial injections, followed by a yearly booster. The vaccine is not 100 percent effective, but these vaccinations are absolutely necessary, especially for all cats that regularly come in contact with other cats.

All cats that test negative for the feline leukemia virus should be vaccinated as early in life as possible. Vaccinating a cat that has tested positive for FeLV is useless in preventing or fighting the virus.

FIP (feline infectious peritonitis)

Q: My veterinarian says my cat has FIP and probably will die. Exactly what is FIP, and how can it be prevented? Are my other cats in danger?

A: Feline infectious peritonitis (FIP) is a very contagious, usually deadly disease, and your other cats are at great risk of becoming infected. However, a vaccination has been developed to help protect them.

There are two forms of the FIP disease. When a cat has the "dry" form of FIP, small inflamed lesions spread throughout the body's organs. The symptoms of this form are vague, usually consisting of persistent, chronic fever, weight loss, depression and neurological signs.

When a cat has the "wet" form of FIP, fluid accumulates in the chest and abdominal cavities. The cat may have fever, weight loss, decreased appetite, depression, abdominal swelling and difficulty breathing.

FIP occurs primarily in cats between six weeks and five years of age, although most victims are younger than two years old. Sometimes pregnant cats are infected, resulting in still-born or weak new-born kittens. Older cats can become more susceptible to FIP when their immune systems weaken.

A veterinarian can run an FIP blood test that will give a very strong indication as to whether or not a cat has FIP.

Cats with the "wet" form of FIP have a characteristic sticky yellow fluid which can be taken from the abdomen or the chest. There is no specific treatment for this ultimately fatal disease, other than general supportive care such as proper nutrition, antibiotics and intravenous fluids to make your pet more comfortable.

The FIP vaccine is given painlessly with a special plastic dropper in the cat's nostril, rather than by needle injection. In addition to the FIP vaccine, proper care of cats and kittens can help prevent the disease. FIP is transmitted by contact with urine, saliva or feces of infected animals. It is very important to minimize the contact that your cat has with strange or obviously ill cats.

Other general preventive measures include keeping your cat's living quarters, litter box, and food and water dishes as clean as possible. Also, be sure your cat is tested for the feline leukemia virus (FeLV) and feline AIDS (FIV), and receives all recommended vaccinations—including the FIP vaccine—during an annual physical examination by your veterinarian.

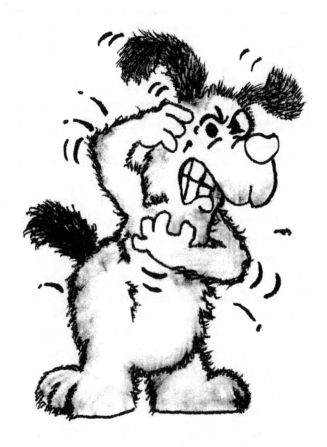

Flea Problems

Q: My dogs are already starting to have flea problems this summer. Isn't there something other than steroid shots and chemical powders that can stop the itching?

A: The key to preventing flea problems is to follow a three-step plan to eliminate fleas from your pets' environment, keep them off each pet and use the proper skin care products to promote beautiful, healthy hair coats.

Step one is to treat your house and yard against fleas. There is no way to win the annual battle against these blood-thirsty little parasites without eliminating them from the environment. For every single flea that you see on your pets, there are hundreds—perhaps thousands—of other fleas and little white worms, or flea larvae, in the surrounding area of your home or yard. Fleas don't live on your pet—they just hop on to take a blood meal.

Professional flea control products vary in quality and toxicity. Consult your veterinarian for a recommendation on what products work the best and are safest for you and your pets. For many pet owners, professional exterminators are the best choice. Others prefer to spray their own yards and flea bomb their homes themselves.

In any case, be sure that the treatment kills not only the adult fleas, but also the flea larvae which otherwise will hatch in a week or two to reinfest the area. Repeated treatments may be necessary.

One non-toxic treatment that is very effective, especially for carpeted areas, consists of borate crystals that actually kill the fleas by desiccating or drying them out.

In addition, vacuum your carpets and furniture thoroughly before the treatment of your home, and throw away the vacuum bag. Use premise spray in hard-to-reach areas. Wash your pet's bedding often.

Step two is to coordinate the extermination effort with baths to eliminate fleas from all of your pets—including all cats. Unfortunately, flea baths don't have residual action and only kill fleas on your pet at the time of the bath. Flea dips have very short-acting residual action. They can dry out the pet's skin and hair coat, and actually may be a cause of itching in some cases.

Your veterinarian can provide a prescription flea control treatment that will keep fleas off your pets for about a month if the environment has been treated effectively. Or, you may choose natural, non-toxic flea control by using products containing Australian tea tree oil.

Step three, after the fleas are under control, is to eliminate itching with the proper choice of hypoallergenic shampoo, moisturizing conditioners and a food supplement that contains marine lipids, borage oil and essential fatty acids added to your pet's diet. These ingredients have natural anti-inflammatory properties which can replace the use of cortisone (steroids) in treating itching caused by flea allergies. (See *Skin Care Products*.)

The effectiveness of using yeast, garlic and B vitamin food supplements to control fleas on pets has long been debated. Many pet owners swear that this remedy is helpful, while others report no noticeable results. University studies have been inconclusive or even contradictory. One theory is that the natural sulfur contained in these ingredients can repel fleas. However, it is important to avoid products that add inappropriate amounts of sulfur because of potential damage to the kidneys.

Limited use of cortisone can be helpful to stop the itch-scratch cycle, but if steroid injections or pills are the only treatment over an extended period of time, serious side-effects can result.

Food Allergies

Q: My cat rubs her face and licks her stomach constantly. Now her hair is coming out in those places. She never seems to stop itching. Could she have a food allergy?

A: Diet and related deficiency of nutrients can definitely affect the condition of the skin and general health of both dogs and cats. Allergic reactions to specific foods also can develop. Food allergies can cause constant itching all year around.

An allergic reaction to food can happen within minutes or hours after the pet eats, or there may be a delayed response that occurs several days later. Most commonly the pet becomes allergic to a food that has been a regular part of its diet for several years.

Food allergies can cause a variety of skin problems, but the major symptom is severe, non-stop itching. Allergic dogs or cats can create so much trauma to the skin that they cause sores, "hot spots" and skin infections. Many pets also develop ear problems and scaly dandruff as a result. Some pets even have related intestinal problems and suffer from vomiting and diarrhea.

To test for food allergy, your cat should be fed a hypoallergenic diet for about three to six weeks. These diets must be individualized for each pet's specific needs to avoid preservatives, colorings, flavorings and foods that the pet has eaten previously.

Switching from one commercial diet to another is not satisfactory because most pet foods contain many of the same ingredients, such as beef, chicken, wheat or corn. Instead, the food allergy diet often will consist of lamb and rice or rabbit and rice.

Consult with your veterinarian about the right hypoallergenic diet for your pet. Remember that cats need an amino acid called taurine in their diets to prevent heart disease.

Food Supplement

Q: My dogs eat a premium quality kibble, but their coats look dry and dull. Should I be adding something to their food?

A: Adding the proper food supplement to your dogs' diet can make a dramatic difference in the appearance of their coats, and also can eliminate excessive shedding, dandruff and dry skin, as well as itching caused by various allergies.

Essential fatty acids and other important nutrients that are critical for healthy skin and hair can be destroyed by heat during the manufacture and storage of most commercial pet foods, including premium pet foods. A lack of these essential fatty acids is one of the major causes of skin problems in dogs and cats, resulting in itching and scratching; dandruff or dry, scaly skin; dry, brittle hair coat; excessive shedding and hair loss; and smelly skin odor.

Dogs and cats cannot produce essential fatty acids in their bodies, but these nutrients easily can be added to the diet each day.

The best pet food supplements contain a combination of borage oil, essential fatty acids and marine lipids (fish oils), as well as vitamins A and E, and lecithin.

Lecithin enables the body to absorb the essential fatty acids naturally without added chemicals. Water soluble food supplements require chemical processing to enable oil and water to mix, and the same absorption benefits can be achieved naturally by adding lecithin to a supplement.

Pets that suffer from pollen allergies and arthritis also can benefit from food supplements that contain fish oils and borage oil. Both marine lipids and borage oil are rich in omega 3, a natural anti-inflammatory ingredient that reduces itching like steroids— but without the side effects.

Products that contain only fish oil or only essential fatty acids or only borage oil do not provide nearly the same benefits as those ingredients used in combination.

Dietary supplements usually take three or four weeks to begin reducing itching and making a noticeable difference in a pet's hair coat. In many cases, the results can be dramatic. Even pets with normal skin and coats can benefit from the added nutrition that the supplements provide.

Foxtails

Q: During a long hike in the country last week, my dog started sneezing. He still sneezes occasionally, and now he has a bloody nose. What could be causing that?

A: Your dog may have sniffed a "foxtail" or other foreign object into one of his nostrils.

Foxtails are those nasty little yellow barbed weeds that cover vacant lots and fields in many areas of the country. They are notorious for clinging to your socks and finding their way into your pet's ears, nose, eyes and between his toes. The foxtails are shaped like arrows with tiny barbs, so they can only move forward, often migrating far into the body. Sometimes foxtails can cause severe infections because they carry bacteria deep into the tissues.

When foxtails are sniffed up the nose, your pet can begin sneezing and even bleeding from the nostrils if the sharp barbs cut into the tissue. In the ears, a foxtail can work its way into the auditory canal, causing infection and possibly even hearing loss. Foxtails between the toes sometimes migrate clear up the leg and into the torso of the animal, or they may travel from the nose all the way to the lungs and abdomen.

Sometimes the initial signs will disappear as the foxtail travels through the various tissues, only to cause other problems later. Foxtails can lodge in tissue inside the body, where an infection or abscess may form. Surgery may be required to remove the foxtail and drain the infected area.

As soon as your pet begins shaking his head, sneezing or limping, take him to a veterinarian to be thoroughly checked before the problem becomes serious.

Your veterinarian may need to use a general anesthesia for direct examination of your dog's nostrils. Medical treatment can range from extracting the foxtail from the affected nose or ear with a special instrument to performing major surgery.

Sometimes a foxtail is not the obvious cause of the symptoms, and X rays or other testing will be needed to rule out problems such as a tumor or bleeding disorder.

Whenever your pet has been running in the grass or weeds, check the ears, eyes, nose and feet for any foxtails that might have been picked up. If possible, discourage your pet from playing in areas such as fields and hills that are covered with foxtails.

Glaucoma

Q: My ten-year-old cockapoo has started to squint all the time. Her right eye seems cloudy and red. Could she be developing an eye problem?

A: Glaucoma is one condition that could cause the symptoms you describe, especially considering the age and breed of your dog. Glaucoma is a disease in which pressure builds in the eye, sometimes leading to blindness.

The eye is constantly producing fluid that circulates in the eye, and this fluid drains back into the bloodstream. When the fluid fails to drain properly, the pressure in the eye increases and—if left untreated—can damage the retina and optic nerve.

Glaucoma is typically seen in middle-aged dogs, especially cocker spaniels and terriers. The most common symptoms are changes in the eye's appearance and in the animal's behavior. Since glaucoma can be very painful, pets may begin to squint, avoid bright lights or look for places to hide. Unfortunately, sometimes there are no signs until the pressure in the animal's eye is very high and the vision already is lost.

The disease may develop over a long period of time or within a few days. Other symptoms can include reddening and inflammation of the white part of the eye, a dilated pupil, and a cloudy blue or white, milky-looking cornea. In advanced cases, the eye may bulge so much that the eyelid cannot cover the eye. This causes the cornea to dry out and ulcers may form. In cats, the only sign may be a dilated pupil and a bulging eye. They rarely show the signs of pain that are seen in dogs with glaucoma.

Nothing can prevent glaucoma, but it usually can be treated medically. Medication can be used to slow the fluid production and increase drainage from the eye. Your pet may be hospitalized for several days during treatment because the dosage of required medication is so critical. After that, the pet owner must treat the animal at home indefinitely.

Surgery often can be an alternative. Cyclocryosurgery allows the veterinarian to freeze the eye's fluid-producing tissue, which will eliminate future buildup of pressure. If the eye must be removed, it can be replaced with a false eye, so your pet will look normal.

Glaucoma is a true medical emergency. If the pressure becomes very high for even a few hours, your pet's sight may be irreversibly lost.

Hairballs

Q: Every once in a while my three-year-old cat gags, makes horrible retching sounds and then vomits. Otherwise, she seems perfectly healthy. Should I be concerned?

A: One of the most common causes of occasional

gagging or vomiting in an apparently healthy cat is a hairball that accumulates in the stomach from licking and gooming. This is especially prevalent in long-haired breeds.

To remedy the problem, try taking half of a teaspoon of petroleum jelly on your finger and putting it on the roof of your cat's mouth each day for a week. This helps lubricate the cat's digestive tract so the hairball can pass out in the stool.

If your cat is finicky and objects to this procedure, there are better-tasting lubricants available from a pet store or your veterinarian. If your cat still refuses to cooperate, or continues having problems, a veterinarian can help.

Heart Attack

Q: My fourteen-year-old cocker spaniel had a heart attack recently and is now on medication. What can I do to help keep her from having another one that might be fatal?

A: Congestive heart failure occurs when a dog's heart is unable to maintain an adequate blood flow and cannot give the body enough oxygen. The options for treatment depend on the exact cause of the problem.

There are many different kinds of heart failure in dogs. Congenital heart disease is an abnormality of the heart at birth. Your veterinarian will check for this condition during the puppy's first exam. Any puppy that doesn't gain weight or grow normally should be checked for heart problems.

Another common heart ailment is due to problems with heart valves. This type of heart failure usually comes on very slowly, and dogs with this condition often can do very well on heart medications for long periods of time.

Another heart problem involves abnormal conduction of the impulses in the heart. This often is seen in older cocker spaniels and dachshunds. Medications can act as a chemical pacemaker in many of these cases.

Heartworm disease has become a more common cause of heart failure in dogs. Check with your veterinarian to determine if you live in a heartworm risk area. Prevention of heartworm-related heart disease is quite easy by giving your dog monthly medication. (See *Heartworm.*)

The first sign of heart disease often is coughing. The heart enlarges to compensate for less efficient pumping of blood and puts pressure on the bronchial tubes.

Another common symptom of heart disease is fatigue or heavy panting after mild exercise.

In heart failure, fluid can build up in the animal's chest or abdomen. The breathing can become very labored, rapid and shallow. The dog may extend its neck in an attempt to get more oxygen. The heart rate may be too fast or slow, the gums may become pale or blue and the blood circulation drops, leading to weakness, collapse and sudden death.

A veterinarian may be able to hear heart murmurs that often are present if your pet is having heart problems. Special tests such as ultrasound, ECG studies and X-rays can help determine the exact causes of the heart disease.

A veterinary heart specialist can even do special dye studies on the heart and its vessels, just like in human medicine.

Treatment of heart problems often includes restricted exercise, heart medications and a special prescription diet that is low in salt and protein.

Surgery may be necessary in some cases.

Heartworm

Q: Should I have my dog tested for heartworm? I used to live in an area where heartworm was a real problem, but here people don't seem as concerned.

A: Heartworm is a deadly disease carried by mosquitoes, and in many parts of the country it has become a serious epidemic. Now the disease is gradually spreading wherever there are mosquitoes.

In many parts of the world, heartworm is the single biggest health problem for dogs.

Dog owners who want to be careful and protect their pets from this spreading, life-threatening disease should ask their veterinarians to test their pets for heartworm. If your dog tests negative, your veterinarian will recommend a simple preventive program, usually consisting of one tablet of medication each month. This not only protects your pet, but helps stop the spread of this disease.

It is very important never to give heartworm medication to dogs that have not been tested or that have tested positive for heartworm because it can make them very sick.

It is particularly critical for any dog that travels to areas where heartworm is a problem to be tested for heartworm and put on a preventive program.

The spread of heartworm begins when a mosquito bites an infected dog. The mosquito withdraws blood containing microscopic immature heartworm, larvae called microfilaria. Inside the mosquito, the microfilaria undergo a series of changes, and within two or three weeks develop into infective larvae. The larvae are then passed into another dog when the mosquito takes its next blood meal.

Continuing their development in the dog, the larvae mature into adult worms in about six months. Adult heartworms are six to ten inches long and collect primarily in the right chambers of the heart and in blood vessels that take blood to the lungs.

Microfilaria are continually released by female heartworms and circulate throughout the dog's body. The adult heartworms cause damage by increasing the work load of the heart and impairing circulation to the lungs, liver and kidneys.

When heartworm begins affecting the dog's heart,

signs include coughing, lack of energy and reduced appetite.

If a blood test for heartworms is positive, the dog usually is given intravenous medication to kill the worms. The dog must be monitored very carefully during this time because it may become very sick as the heartworms die.

Symptoms of heartworm disease usually are not evident until after major organs have been damaged. This makes early detection and prevention very important.

Hereditary Problems

Q: My daughter wants to get a miniature poodle, but I've heard that they have a lot of medical problems. Is that true?

A: Most purebred dogs are more susceptible to inherited defects than mixed breeds, and miniature poodles are no exception. Always be sure to ask your veterinarian to thoroughly examine any pet before the purchase or adoption is finalized so that you know what to expect.

Another good way to help predict your pet's future health is to meet the mother and father. If they are healthy, well-behaved animals, your dog is more likely to share those characteristics.

Miniature poodles can be wonderful, loving pets. However, they sometimes carry abnormal genes that cause a variety of problems, including a defect in the arteries near the heart, unusually short leg bones, brittle bones, dislocated shoulders or kneecaps, degeneration of the retina, and bladder stones.

Miniature and toy poodles also can suffer from epilepsy, diabetes and loss of insulation around the nerves and spinal cord.

In addition, this breed often is afflicted with skin allergies, ear problems and plugged tear ducts.

These skin problems can result from allergies to fleas, pollen, food or the chemicals used in many shampoos. The solution often is a program that combines a proper diet supplemented with omega 3 from marine lipids, a hypoallergenic shampoo and an effective flea control program.

The ear problems usually result from hair that grows down into the ear canal and causes chronic inflammation unless it is pulled out. This is particularly troublesome if the dog has allergies that make the ear canal very sensitive. Your veterinarian can remove the ear hair and recommend a soothing ear washing and drying solution to use on a regular basis to prevent more serious ear problems.

Plugged tear ducts cause secretions from the eyes to run from the corners of the eyes, often causing dark, moist stains on the poodle's face.

Most inherited defects can be treated by your veterinarian—either medically, nutritionally or surgically—to improve the quality of your pet's life.

Hernia (umbilical)

Q: I have a new puppy with a little swelling on her tummy by her bellybutton. She seems to feel fine. Should I be worried?

A: A slight swelling on the abdomen of a puppy could be the symptom of a condition called an umbilical hernia. Such hernias usually are not serious, but you should have your puppy examined by a veterinarian to be sure.

The umbilical hernia is an opening that develops in the wall of the abdomen where the umbilical cord was attached. When the muscles don't grow together properly, the hernia occurs.

The exact cause of umbilical hernias isn't known. They may be inherited defects or perhaps the result of trauma to the umbilical cord during birth. In some cases, the mother pulls too hard on the cord, and in other cases the cord may be cut too short.

Umbilical hernias are more common in dogs than in cats.

Most umbilical hernias will not have to be repaired immediately and can be surgically corrected when your pet is old enough to be spayed or neutered. However, it is important to watch the umbilical hernia in case complications develop.

For example, if your pet's intestines should enter through the hole in the abdominal wall and strangulate, the umbilical hernia condition becomes an

emergency. The hernia may contract around the pro-
truding intestine, preventing it from returning into
the abdominal cavity, cutting off the blood supply.
In this case, surgery should be performed immediately.

Hernias sometimes develop in the groin area. The
intestines can bulge through these inguinal hernias,
resulting in severe discomfort and causing the same
kinds of medical problems as umbilical hernias.

Hip Dysplasia

**Q: My dog has hip dysplasia. I understand
there may be some new research developments
that could cure this problem. What can you tell
me about that?**

A: Hip dysplasia, usually a hereditary disease,
causes painful arthritis in the hips, primarily in large
breed or fast-growing dogs. Veterinarians are able
to make the victims of hip dysplasia more comfortable with medication, but other cases may require
surgery, including a hip replacement.

The hip joint is a ball and socket joint, with the
head of the thigh bone as the ball that fits into the
socket formed by the pelvic bones coming together.
In some dogs, the tissues that support this joint are
loose, allowing too much movement of the bone in
the socket. This abnormal movement eventually
causes destruction of the joint. The damaged joint

and the arthritis that follows cause the pain and lameness of hip dysplasia.

Often the first sign of hip dysplasia will be a change in the normal gait of a young dog—the result of looseness in the joint. Lameness may occur after exercise. As the dog ages, degenerative arthritis develops in the hips, causing pain and stiffness.

Early stages of hip dysplasia can be treated with rest and pain medications such as aspirin. Be sure to consult your veterinarian about the proper type of pain medication and dosage because some common pain medications that are appropriate for humans can be dangerous for dogs.

More severe arthritis in the hip joint may require anti-inflammatory drugs such as cortisone. Food supplements with marine lipids can act as a natural anti-inflammatory ingredient and give significant relief to dogs with arthritis in the hip joint.

Conscientious breeders have been working for years to limit hip dysplasia by selective breeding. X rays can reveal dysplasia in prospective breeding animals, and those pets should be spayed or neutered to prevent the disease from being passed on to their puppies.

Some large breed dogs are predisposed toward hip dysplasia. Owners of large dogs should have both potential parents X-rayed for hip dysplasia because the problem may not show up until an animal is two years old or older.

"Hot Spots"

Q: My dog suffers from allergies to fleas and pollen. She chews herself raw. How can I treat the "hot spots" and stop the itching?

A: The "hot spots" that result when your animal licks and chews herself are usually secondary bacterial infections that develop due to the damage that has been done to the skin.

A hot spot can start off looking like a little red area the size of a dime, and quickly spread to become a huge, oozing lesion the size of your hand by the end of the day. Hot spots can be very painful for your pet and should get immediate attention. In addition, it is very important to control the underlying problem—often allergies to fleas, pollen or food that cause the itching.

Veterinarians typically prescribe cortisone, an anti-inflammatory steroid, to stop the itch-scratch cycle of the allergy, and antibiotics to fight the infection. Steroids can have serious side effects if given regularly over an extended period of time.

Unfortunately, some topical sprays prescribed to treat hot spots contain alcohol, lidocain, hydrocortisone, or other harsh chemical ingredients that can damage, burn or dry out your pet's skin.

A more natural approach is almost always more effective. For example, skin care products for pets that contain tea tree oil, chamomile and aloe vera can clear up most hot spots in just a few days. Australian tea tree oil is a natural healing ingredient that has been used for centuries by aborigines to reduce inflammation and itching, treat infections, and repel fleas, flies, ticks and mosquitoes. Aloe vera and chamomile are soothing ingredients to reduce pain and promote healing.

Even though hot spots can be eliminated, the problem will recur unless the source of the allergy is controlled. A wide range of flea control products are available, but it is important to remember that you must have a total plan to eliminate fleas. You must eliminate fleas on all pets in the household, eliminate fleas and flea larvae in the house, and eliminate fleas in the outside yard or kennel.

Veterinary clinic and pet store staff usually are trained to recommend flea control products and extermination services that suit your individual situation. Some people prefer a natural, environmentally friendly approach to flea control, while others want to be very aggressive about eliminating the pesky little parasites, even if that means using some potent pesticides.

Pets with pollen allergies can be skin tested by a veterinarian and hyposensitized with allergen injections. Or a food supplement containing marine lipids, essential fatty acids and borage oil can be added to their diets. (See *Skin Care Products*.)

Hot Weather

Q: My pets always seem to get into trouble during hot weather and end up having to go to the vet. What precautions can I take?

A: The hot summer months present some special hazards for pets, whether they are playing in the park, swimming in the pool, romping at the beach or just riding around in the family car. Here are some common dangers to avoid:

• Cars parked in the sun on a hot day can be ovens for pets. Never leave your dog or cat in a closed car during the heat of the day. Even a few minutes can raise the temperature enough to cause heatstroke that could be fatal to your pet.

• Many dogs enjoy swimming in the ocean, but the salt water can make animals seriously ill if they drink too much. Always have plenty of fresh drinking water available. Pets that swim in salt water also should be rinsed off with clear water to avoid skin problems.

• Pool chemicals are necessary to keep your pool sanitary, but if your pet drinks undiluted chlorine, severe acid burns can result. Be sure your pet knows how to get out of the pool before allowing a swim. Also, clean and dry your pet's ear canals after each swim to prevent painful ear infections and rinse the coat to help avoid skin problems

• Foxtails, grass awns and weed seeds, and stickers of various kinds can catch in your pet's hair.

Some burrow right into the skin or enter eyes, ears, nostrils or between the toes. Careful daily grooming provides a chance to check for these problems, which sometimes result in serious infections.

• "Hot spots" are actually a form of moist infection, often caused by scratching or biting at fleas, or itching and chewing because of pollen allergies. Daily grooming can help to detect a hot spot in the early stages. Flea control, of course, is an absolute necessity during the summer in most areas.

• Sunburn isn't just for humans. White cats and dogs or animals with large pink areas around the nose also can burn. And, if your pet has a fresh, short haircut, be sure to keep the animal out of the sun until protective hair grows out again. Some No. 15 SPF (or higher) waterproof sun block can protect the exposed areas. Even if your pet licks it off, some will soak into the layers of the skin and help prevent sun damage and skin cancer.

Hyperactive Cat

Q: My nine-year-old cat has always had a good appetite, but recently she started eating more and losing weight. She also paces and seems nervous. What could be wrong?

A: Older cats can develop a number of medical problems with the symptoms that you describe, including kidney failure, diabetes, different types of cancer and hyperthyroidism.

The possibility of a hyperactive thyroid gland should be considered in any middle-aged or older cat showing signs of hyperactivity, nervousness, weight loss, increased appetite, increased water consumption, hair loss, vomiting or diarrhea.

Since the thyroid gland controls the metabolism of every single cell in the body, an abnormal increase in the thyroid activity affects many different systems of the body.

Laboratory screening tests should include a complete blood count (CBC), blood chemistry panel, thyroid hormone test and urinalysis. These tests are not only important to diagnose hyperthyroidism, but to rule out other disorders common in older cats.

Testing multiple blood samples for thyroid hormone on different days might be necessary to make a diagnosis because levels vary over a period of time. In rare cases, a thyroid imaging scan may be appropriate.

There are three ways to treat hyperthyroidism. Medication often is used to destroy the thyroid tissue, but surgery sometimes is an option. In a few cases, treatment with radioactive iodine also has been used for cats that are suffering from hyperthyroidism.

Each method has advantages and disadvantages which should be discussed with your veterinarian. If hyperthyroidism is left untreated, a cat eventually will become severely emaciated, with serious organ damage and a high risk of heart failure.

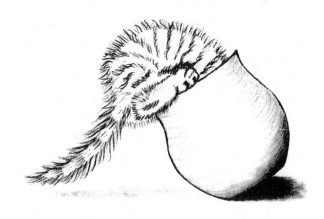

Hypothyroidism

Q: I have an overweight golden retriever that has dry, flaking skin and hair loss. My veterinarian thinks she might be hypothyroid. Can you explain how that is treated?

Hypothyroidism is a common hereditary disease in dogs. The thyroid gland is like a thermostat that controls the metabolism of cells throughout the body, including the skin and hair.

Often dogs that are hypothyroid have dull, dry brittle hair coats, a slow metabolism, are lethargic and may suffer from fatigue. They tend to gain weight easily.

Hypothyroidism also may cause excessive shedding, hair loss in a symmetrical pattern, dry scaling dandruff, oily scaling dandruff, skin infections, and a "sad dog" look, with sleepy or droopy eyes and puffy skin that results in a tragic facial expression. The skin often becomes hyperpigmentated so that it looks black.

Hypothyroidism also can present a wide variety of other symptoms, including a slow heart rate and depressed immune system. As a result, veterinarians sometimes call it "the great impersonator."

Your veterinarian can test your dog's thyroid. If there is a problem, thyroid medication can make a dramatic difference. In addition, medicated bathing, coat conditioning, and the addition of certain essential fatty acids to the diet are all very important for healing the hypothyroid dog.

If laboratory tests indicate that your dog is hypothyroid, medication given daily in appropriate doses often clears up the abnormalities caused by low thyroid function within about three months. A post-pill test four to six weeks after medication is started will determine if the proper dosage of thyroid is being given.

Hypothyroid dogs can live normal, active lives, but they must always stay on medication to compensate for their inability to produce proper levels of thyroid.

In addition to the medication, hypothyroid dogs should have a healthful diet to provide the proper nutrients for the body to heal. Antibiotics often are prescribed to treat skin infections. Medicated bathing and coat conditioning are essential to remove the dead skin and falling hairs, and to keep new skin and hair healthy.

Itching and Scratching

Q: I have a little dog that itches all the time. She chews her paws and has lost a lot of hair on her back above her tail from scratching. What is causing that?

A: Itching and scratching are often caused by combinations of allergies, which can make specific diagnosis and treatment especially challenging for veterinarians.

Itching can be caused by an allergy to fleas (flea allergy dermatitis), pollens, dust and other particles in the air (inhalent allergies), foods (food allergy dermatitis), and substances that touch the skin (contact allergy dermatitis).

Flea allergies are the most common. Pets that suffer from flea bites are actually hypersensitive to the saliva that the flea injects into the animal's skin when it takes a blood meal. After the flea bites, a small red bump develops. If the animal is allergic to the flea's saliva, itching will result. One flea bite can set off an allergic reaction that lasts for two weeks. Loss of hair from scratching on the back above the tail is a common symptom. Pollen and dust allergies also are common. People react to inhaled allergies by developing respiratory signs such as sneezing, hay fever and asthma. Most allergic dogs itch and scratch instead. Pollen allergies usually begin as a seasonal problem, but as time passes the pet becomes more and more allergic, and the allergy can be present all year long. Chewing the front paws and rubbing the face are common symptoms.

Food allergies are not as common, but if your pet is allergic to a certain ingredient in the diet, severe itching and scratching can result. Some of the most common foods that cause allergies in dogs are beef, wheat and corn, but almost any food can cause the problem. Even food dyes and other additives can trigger an allergic reaction in some pets. Food allergies last as long as your pet is exposed to the offending food.

Contact allergies usually affect the areas of the body that are less protected by hair, such as the lower abdomen. Whenever sensitive skin comes in contact with grass, for example, a red, inflamed rash and itching can result.

Frequently dogs with allergies develop secondary skin problems, such as dandruff, hair loss and infections.

Consult a veterinarian to determine which problem or combination of problems is causing your dog to itch and scratch.

"Junk food"

Q: My dog loves junk food. He tries to steal anything with chocolate in it and begs for ice cream. Will that hurt him?

A: Most junk food and desserts are loaded with fat, sugar, salt, artificial colorings and preservatives. These are empty calories that can lead to health problems such as diabetes, pancreatitis and obesity.

Chocolate acts as a poison for dogs because they cannot excrete the theobromine or caffeine. Milk chocolate is less toxic because the caffeine levels are lower than with baker's chocolate, which is very concentrated. Only 2 or 3 ounces of baker's chocolate can be fatal to a 20-pound dog.

The most commonly reported cause of chocolate toxicity is from dogs sampling candy that the owners have left out. Holidays always produce many unfortunate cases of chocolate poisoning in dogs.

Caffeine, one of the most common ingredients in our daily diets, can cause severe medical problems for dogs. Caffeine is found in chocolate, coffee, soft drinks and various medications.

Caffeine is very toxic to dogs and can be lethal. Symptoms of caffeine poisoning include excessive panting, extreme excitability, abnormally fast heart rate, tremors, convulsions and elevated temperature. Sometimes the stimulating effect of caffeine is so great on the central nervous system that cardiac arrest results and emergency medical treatment cannot save the animal.

Resist the temptation to share junk food with your dog. Remarkably, there are even some dog treats on the market that contain both sugar and chocolate. Be sure to read the labels.

If you need to give your pet a treat, try fresh fruits

or vegetables (many dogs love them!), or an all-natural dog biscuit that is free of hydrogenated fats, salt and artificial colorings.

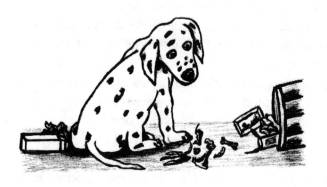

Kennel Cough

Q: The kennel that keeps our dogs when we go on vacation requires a vaccination that is given in the nose. Is it really necessary?

A: The bordetella vaccination, which helps guard your pet against kennel cough, is now given by putting drops into the dog's nostril, rather than by injection. It is painless and very effective.

Kennel cough, or infectious tracheobronchitis, is an upper-respiratory disease that is caused by a combination of a virus (parainfluenza) and a bacteria (bordetella).

Kennel cough is widespread and quite contagious

among unvaccinated dogs that are boarded in kennels. Dogs also can pick up the disease at pet shows, grooming shops, public parks, veterinary clinics or other places where dogs are in close contact with each other.

Kennel cough starts as a slight, dry, hacking cough and often develops into a severe cough. It usually is accompanied by sneezing, nasal discharge and sometimes vomiting. Kennel cough is spread through the air, much like a common cold or influenza is spread among people.

A mild case of kennel cough usually will affect your dog about as long as a heavy cold might affect you. However, dogs with severe cases often have a fever and reduced appetite. If not properly treated, pneumonia might develop. Veterinarians use antibiotics and cough suppressants to treat the disease.

Dogs should be vaccinated once a year to be protected against kennel cough. The bordetella vaccine works within forty-eight hours and allows people to have their dogs vaccinated just a few days before they drop them off at the kennel.

Be sure the kennel staff knows which veterinary clinic has your pet's medical records and what you want done in case of a medical emergency. Also, it is very important that your dog is current on all other vaccinations, including the distemper combination (DHLP), parvo, corona and rabies. In addition, a thorough physical examination by a veterinarian before boarding can help detect serious medical problems that otherwise might develop when you are away.

Kidney Problems

Q: My veterinarian says that my dog has severe kidney problems. What causes that and how should it be treated?

A: The kidneys act as a blood filtration system, eliminating toxins from the body. Kidney disease can be caused by a wide range of factors, including cancer, injuries, infections, parasites, cysts, kidney stones and other diseases.

The kidneys also regulate and balance body fluids. Urine formed in the two kidneys is delivered to the bladder by the ureters. Urine is stored in the bladder until it gets full. When the bladder contracts, the urine is emptied out of the body through the urethra.

One kidney can take over the job, but if both kidneys become diseased or injured, kidney failure results.

It is common for bacteria to cause a bladder infection. This can lead to a serious urinary tract infection if the bacteria backs up into the kidneys.

Symptoms of kidney disease can include increased frequency of urination, greater consumption of water, bloody or cloudy urine, straining to urinate, lack of appetite, vomiting, depression and anemia.

Your veterinarian can diagnose kidney disease by running blood tests that will show anemia or toxins in the blood. X-rays may show stones or tumors in the kidneys, or reveal that a kidney is bigger or smaller than normal. A special dye also may be used to outline the kidneys and bladder to show any obstructions to the flow of urine.

Treatment of kidney disease depends on the degree of damage. Sometimes all that is required is a special diet to lower protein levels that result in the buildup of toxins.

However, if your veterinarian detects a high level of toxins in the bloodstream, your pet may be suffering from uremia. This is a medical emergency. Treatment will include intravenous fluids to flush out the toxins, antibiotics for infection and a strict prescription diet.

Kidney transplants and kidney dialysis like that used for human patients are not readily available for pets.

Knee Injury

Q: My Labrador retriever twisted one of his hind legs while we were hiking. Now he is limping, and the vet says the ligament in his knee is broken. Can you explain?

A: The most frequent knee injury in dogs is the rupture of the cranial cruciate ligament. This results in instability of the knee joint because it helps connect the upper leg bone (the femur) to the lower leg bone (the tibia).

When the cranial cruciate ligament is broken, the knee becomes very "loose," meaning that there is abnormal movement of the knee joint. This condition can result in pain, lameness and eventually arthritis in the joint.

Your veterinarian can tell if the cranial cruciate ligament is ruptured by manipulating the knee and feeling for excessive looseness and movement of the leg bones backward and forward. This movement is called the anterior drawer sign.

The damage can be surgically repaired by using a section of a tendon in the knee to create a new cranial cruciate ligament. This piece of tendon is actually grafted to both the upper leg bone and the lower leg bone to hold them in place in the same way the damaged cranial cruciate ligament did before it ruptured. The ends of the piece of tendon are attached to the leg bones with surgical screws.

At first the graft is weak, but as the months pass it becomes stronger and stronger. In time, most dogs that have this surgery recover completely and lead comfortable, active lives. However, they still can develop some arthritic changes in the knee joint as they grow older.

Medium to large breed dogs are more prone to knee injuries. Often the rupture of the cranial cruciate ligament is the result of trauma caused by hyperextension or abnormal rotation of the knee.

Laboratory Tests

Q: What kind of lab tests do you recommend when I take my dog in for her annual physical exam? She is nine-years-old and seems to be in pretty good health.

A: Routine physical exams for people almost always include blood work and a urinalysis, and the physician also often suggests an ECG and X rays to support conclusions about the health of the patient. Since dogs and cats can't comment on how they feel, such tests can be even more helpful for a veterinarian. As dogs and cats get older, they often experience two types of changes with increasing frequency. First, age-related changes in vision and hearing are normal and develop in most animals. Second, diseases such as cancer, arthritis, diabetes, and heart, liver or kidney problems occur with greater frequency. Most of the medical problems in this second category can be treated successfully if they are diagnosed early.

Blood panels can give important information about how the liver, kidneys, heart, pancreas and other organs are functioning. A complete blood count (CBC) can help in the diagnosis of bacterial and viral infections, anemia, clotting problems and cancers.

A urinalysis gives an indication of how the kidneys are functioning and also serves as an all-purpose screen for systemic disease. An electrocardiogram (ECG) can help your veterinarian assess your pet's heart and detect any irregular, slow or weak heartbeat.

X-rays can help uncover changes such as enlargements or reductions in organ size, accumulation of fluid, presence of tumors, arthritic changes in joints, and the presence of bladder stones.

Ultrasound can be very valuable in diagnosing everything from pregnancies to tumors.

Consultation about a diet that meets your pet's changing nutritional needs also is a very important part of any thorough checkup.

In addition to the physical exam and appropriate tests, your pet's basic health care program should include vaccinations, fecal exams to check for parasites, an annual dentistry and regular heartworm tests if you live in an area where any mosquitoes are present.

Leg Inflammation

Q: My one-year-old German shepherd keeps getting lame in different legs. Sometimes the limp will go away and then come back. What could be wrong?

A: Your dog could be suffering from a disease called panosteitis that occurs most often in adolescent large and giant breed dogs—especially German shepherds and Dobermans. The condition is an inflammation of the long bones in the legs.

The disease begins with a decreased density in the middle cavity of the bone in the region where the bone gets its blood supply. Researchers do not know what causes this change.

After the density decreases, there is an increase in bony tissue. Your veterinarian usually can first notice the changes in an X-ray taken about 10–14 days after the dog becomes lame.

The discomfort that is caused by panosteitis often causes dogs to shift their weight on different legs, so they may limp first on one leg, then another. The disease also commonly comes in cycles, which explains the unusual pattern of the symptoms that you described.

Other signs of panosteitis can include fever, lack of appetite, depression and just feeling sick. Male dogs are more commonly affected than females.

The disease often is painful when the tissues over the affected areas are touched.

Fortunately, this medical problem is not life threatening. Restricted activity and possibly a pain reliever recommended by your veterinarian will make your pet more comfortable, but with this disease, the most effective medicine is simply the passing of time. Typically, your pet will be back to normal in about two to four months.

Leg Injuries

Q: I adopted a pair of calico kittens that had been running wild. One of them has deformed front legs. They bow out, and her feet turn in. Can that be corrected?

A: Trauma to the front legs, perhaps caused by jumping from a high place, can result in problems with the growing bones in kittens or puppies.

The long bones of the legs grow at areas called growth plates. If the growth plate areas are damaged, they can prematurely stop the growth of the bones. This can result in bowing of the long bones and abnormal rotation of the foot, like the condition you describe in your cat. In addition to a leg deformity, a related arthritic condition may develop in some of the animal's joints.

Nutritional deficiencies also can severely affect the bones and their ability to grow normally. A young animal has soft bones with a lot of cartilage. Part of the growing process involves calcification in the bones. If the young animal doesn't have a balanced diet, the bone cannot calcify properly.

An all-meat diet could be very harmful. Meat is very high in phosphorus. If the phosphorus level is too high and there is not an adequate supply of calcium in the diet, the body will pull calcium out of the bones. As a result, the bones will become soft and can even develop folds or "folding fractures." This is a desperate situation for a young animal trying to form healthy bones.

Your calico kitten could be suffering the effects of either trauma to the legs, nutritional deficiency, or both. The first step is for X-rays to be taken by a veterinarian to find out exactly what her bone structure looks like. Surgical correction may be recommended. Be sure your pet is on a high quality, balanced diet. Adding meat to a good commercial pet food only throws off the calcium-phosphorus ratio.

Liver Disease

Q: My Westy has been diagnosed as having liver disease. Can you explain how she got it and what can be done?

A: Some breeds of dogs, including West Highland white terriers, don't excrete copper from their systems the way they should, and this can lead to liver disease. More common causes for other breeds are viral and bacterial infections, poisonous substances eaten by the pet, and restricted blood flow to the liver as a result of heart disease or congenital abnormality.

The liver is the largest gland in your dog's body, and serves many complex functions. As a result, many medical disorders can cause liver problems.

The most common signs of liver disease in dogs and cats include lack of appetite and weight loss, depression, yellowing of the gums or the whites of the eyes, increased thirst and dark-colored urine.

Other signs of illness associated with problems involving the liver can include pale gums, fluid buildup in the abdomen and abnormal bleeding. Your pet's abdomen may become enlarged as a result of the accumulation of fluid and enlargement of the liver.

These symptoms, which may appear quickly or develop slowly, also could be signs of a wide range of other medical problems, so it is important to take your pet to a veterinarian for a complete physical exam.

Cats that refuse to eat for two or three days could be suffering from a liver problem called hepatic lipidosis, in which fat builds up to a dangerously high level in the liver. The fat continues to accumulate until it overwhelms the liver's ability to function properly.

Your veterinarian will examine your pet's tongue and gums for the yellowing associated with jaundice, and will feel the abdomen for abnormalities. A blood test will be helpful, since certain enzymes in the blood usually are elevated during liver disease. A liver biopsy also might be recommended.

Treatment of liver disease depends on what caused the initial damage. If your pet has an infection, antibiotics usually are appropriate. If the damage has resulted from poison or too much copper in the system hospitalization and good nursing care will be the main therapy. In all cases, a proper diet recommended by your veterinarian will be very important.

The liver has an excellent capacity to regenerate its cells, so chances are good for recovery when the problem is diagnosed early and treated properly.

Lyme Disease

Q: Every time I take my dogs on a hike in the hills they come home loaded with ticks. How common is Lyme disease? Should I take precautions?

A: Ticks are parasites that can transmit a variety of diseases to pets and humans, including Lyme disease, one of the fastest spreading diseases in North America. A vaccine against Lyme disease is now available. All dogs that live or travel in areas where Lyme disease has been reported should be vaccinated.

The spiral-shaped Lyme disease bacteria, carried by the small deer tick, cause flu-like symptoms, including fatigue, headache and sometimes a skin rash in people. If left untreated, heart, nerve and joint problems can develop.

Pets with Lyme disease often have a sudden onset of severe depression with hot, swollen, painful joints and a strong reluctance to move. In addition, they usually begin to show signs of fever, fatigue, enlarged spleen, swollen lymph nodes and lack of appetite. The most common diagnostic symptom in animals is lameness from acutely inflamed joints.

Veterinarians can confirm Lyme disease using laboratory tests, but a positive result only indicates that the pet has been exposed to the organism that carries the disease at some point in time. Many of the animals that test positive never develop the symptoms of the disease.

If treatment with antibiotics is started early enough, all symptoms of Lyme disease typically can be eliminated within forty-eight hours. However, it is important that the medication be given for a full 10–14 day period to avoid recurrence. Some pets, however, take months to recover, and some bacteria are becoming resistant to medication.

Pets can't transmit Lyme disease to humans, but be careful when removing ticks from your animals. Use tweezers to grasp the tick's head and body and pull it away from your pet's skin. Avoid squashing the tick with your fingers because you might become infected if Lyme disease bacteria are present. Disinfect the bite area with alcohol.

If your pet has many ticks, or if you don't want to deal with the nasty little parasites, bring your animal to a veterinarian so experienced staff can remove the ticks and recommend a tick repellent with residual action to prevent recurrence.

Tick populations are largest during the summer months, and ticks are more prevalent in thick brush and wooded hillsides or canyon areas. Dogs are more likely than cats to get Lyme disease, and horses also can become infected.

Mange (demodex)

Q: I have a puppy that is losing hair in patches all over her body. She doesn't itch much. What could be causing that?

A: An inherited skin disease called demodectic mange can cause the symptoms that you describe, and often is seen in young dogs.

Demodex, or red mange, is caused by a microscopic mite that looks like a little cigar with eight legs. A few demodex mites normally are found at the base of some hairs of both pets and humans. But a medical problem arises when a hereditary defect in the animal's immune system allows the mites to multiply rapidly. The result is hair loss in patches where the mites are most abundant, often accompanied by inflammation and infection of the skin.

Demodectic mange by itself is not an itchy skin disease, but itching may result because of skin infection and related irritation.

Demodectic mange may start on the face or forelegs, stay localized in several small areas and then disappear without treatment. However, if the areas of hair loss start to spread and become infected, this is called "generalized demodectic mange," and treatment should not be delayed.

First, a skin scraping is necessary to determine whether an abnormal number of mites are present on the animal. If bacterial infection is severe, blood tests and cultures of the pus may be necessary to determine the best antibiotic. The tests also show if there are other related problems, such as low thyroid function and anemia.

Medicated baths and special dips are needed, usually over a period of several months, to kill the mites. The hair loss in the affected areas will look worse when the mites are dying, before the condition improves. The immune systems of some dogs are so weak that they never can be cured completely, but most cases of demodectic mange can be controlled very effectively.

Since demodectic mange is a hereditary disease, affected animals should never be bred.

Mating

Q: Our seven-month-old female cat is howling constantly, trying to escape outdoors and rolling around on the floor! She is driving us crazy! What could be wrong with her?

A: If your cat has not been spayed, one possibility is that she is in heat. Cats reach breeding age at six to eleven months of age, and the behavior that you describe is typical.

Estrus (heat) lasts five to six days if your cat does

not mate with a male. She will then be out of heat for the next two to three weeks before the cycle repeats itself. Cats tend to have one breeding season lasting from January to March and another from June to July, during which time they go through repeated cycles unless they are bred or spayed. Feline pregnancies last an average of about two months.

The spay surgery is actually an ovariohysterectomy. If you plan to breed your cat, you should wait until the second or third estrus to allow your cat to mature and gain weight. Due to the large number of unwanted and homeless pets, it would be best to have your cat spayed as soon as possible—usually at about six months of age—to prevent pregnancy if you don't want her to have kittens.

Cats also have less chance of developing mammary tumors as they grow older if they are spayed before one year of age.

Neutering of male pets is essential to control the population of unwanted puppies and kittens. This basic surgical procedure cuts down on injuries related to roaming and fighting, and reduces the risk of being exposed to contagious diseases like FIP, FeLV and feline AIDS. The surgery also decreases the risk of prostatitis, as well as testicular and prostatic cancers.

Dogs reach breeding age at six to twelve months of age. Smaller breeds are ready for breeding earlier than larger breeds because they attain their adult body weight faster.

Dogs have a 7–10 day pre-heat period during

which there is a spotty, bloody vaginal discharge. The female will not allow the male to breed her during this time. Estrus, or the actual heat, lasts an average of seven to nine days.

The dog cycles into heat twice a year at seven- to eight-month intervals, depending on the breed. The basenji is an exception, coming into heat only once each year, usually in the fall.

The dog has no breeding season like the cat, although there is a slight increase in the number of females coming into heat during the late winter and spring months. Pregnancy typically lasts about two months. In older dogs, the interval between heats and the length of pregnancy both increase, and the litter size decreases.

Multi-toed Cats

Q: My kitten has extra-large feet with more toes than normal. Will she need special care? Can surgery correct this problem?

A: Cats with extra toes are called polydactyls, and the deformity is not a handicap at all. Quite the contrary, most multi-toed cats have excellent dexterity and often are quite adept at hunting and opening doors or bags of cat food.

The only special care your kitty will need is some extra love for every single toe. Owners of multi-toed cats claim that their pets have very unique personality traits, and that they express more emotions than cats with normal toes by caressing or "making muffins" with their feet.

Polydactylic cats don't always have the same number of toes on all four feet. In fact, some have a different number on each paw. For example, a cat might have four toes on one paw, five on another and seven on the other two feet. Some cats also have webbed toes or toes that look like thumbs.

A normal cat has four toes on each foot with a pad and nail associated with each one.

Having extra toes is a dominant inherited condition. A polydactyl cat mated to a cat with regular toes usually will produce a litter of half extra-toed kittens and half regular-toed kittens.

Nervous Grooming

Q: Since we brought our new baby home, my cat has been licking herself constantly. Now she is getting bald spots on her sides. Could she be jealous of the baby?

A: There are many possible reasons for excessive grooming, including your suggestion that your cat is jealous because of lack of attention. Changes in your cat's routine or environment (such as new pets, new human babies, overcrowding or moving to a new home) can result in the type of licking that you describe. Psychogenic licking is most common in more emotional breeds, such as Siamese, Burmese, Himalayan and Abyssinians.

Usually cats that are nervous groomers will repeatedly lick one or two areas, often on a leg, side or abdomen. You may notice broken hairs and some patches of hair loss with normal skin showing. Other cats will not only lick off the hair, but also create red, raw, open sores. Sometimes artistic bald stripes will appear down the middle of the cat's back or around the inner thighs, abdominal or genital areas.

Some cats are "closet groomers," and their owners have no idea how the abnormal hair loss and sore spots are occurring.

Samples of your cat's hair can be studied under a microscope to determine if they have been broken off, rather than just falling out. Bald areas on cats that are neurotic groomers are always within reach of the pet's mouth, and other areas of hair and skin appear normal. Often there is a very real underlying cause such as allergies to fleas, foods or pollen. Other types of skin problems which can have similar hair-loss patterns can be ruled out by your veterinarian through various tests such as skin scrapings, fungal cultures, food elimination diets and skin testing.

Medications such as tranquilizers can be used to break the bad habit of excessive grooming, but the underlying cause of the behavior should be identified and eliminated. Some temperamental cats may need to take medication for the rest of their lives to control the behavior. Other cats can be completely cured.

New Kittens

Q: My cat is pregnant, and I'm getting nervous about what will happen when she gives birth. What do I need to know?

A: About two weeks before giving birth, the mother cat should be introduced to a whelping box—a warm, dimly lit box in a familiar environment.

About two or three days before the birth, the mother cat may lose her appetite and her vulva may appear swollen. You also might notice a slight discharge from the area.

The mother cat usually becomes restless as she goes into labor. When strong contractions begin, she typically will lie on her side and start licking herself, purring and groaning.

After awhile, the mother cat's water bag will appear and either break by itself or be broken by her. Soon the head of the first kitten will appear enclosed in the amniotic sac. The mother cat will break the sac, lick the kitten and bite off the umbilical cord.

If the mother cat fails, you can break the amniotic sac and rub the kitten briskly but gently until it begins breathing. Then return the newborn kitten to the mother cat. The placenta, or afterbirth, usually is eaten by the mother cat.

Litters can vary from one kitten to eight or more. The time between births varies from fifteen minutes to more than an hour.

Kittens are born with their eyes and ear canals closed. Since they can neither see nor hear, they depend solely on their mother for nourishment, warmth and protection. For the first three critical days, the kittens should be kept with the mother cat in the whelping box and not be disturbed. Huddling with the mother cat has a calming effect on the kittens, and they spend most of their time nursing.

It is important for you to keep a close watch on newborn kittens to make sure each is getting a fair share of milk and is showing no sign of illness. It is also important to resist the temptation to handle kittens until they are several days old. Don't change the soiled blanket in the maternity box until about three days after the kittens are born.

Chilling is a frequent cause of kitten death because young cats can't regulate their own body temperatures. It is critical that the whelping box be kept at about 85 degrees. Be careful not to overheat or burn the kittens, and provide an area for escape from constant heat and light.

Kittens have a well-developed sense of smell, which helps them find their mother's nipple for nursing. During the first twenty-four hours, a thin, milk-like substance called colostrum is produced, which is very rich in antibodies that protect kittens against diseases for the first few weeks. By three days of age, each kitten selects a preferred nipple. Nipple preference assures the milk production, because if a gland is not suckled for three days, milk will no longer be produced. "Milk tread" is the rhythmic alternating movement of the kitten's forepaws against the gland, which helps the flow of milk.

Young kittens cannot urinate or defecate until they are about three weeks old without stimulation by the mother cat licking their genital regions.

When the kittens are ten to fourteen days old, they open their eyes and also begin to hear sounds.

Kittens are born with some instincts but also learn by observing their mothers. Runts in a normal litter can have decreased learning ability because of lack of nutrition and may suffer psychological problems because of intimidation by other littermates.

Most kittens double their weight in the first week and triple their weight in the second week. Weaning takes place gradually, starting at about 4 weeks of age, and usually is complete by 8 to 10 weeks. During this time, the kitten makes a transition from nursing to eating solid food.

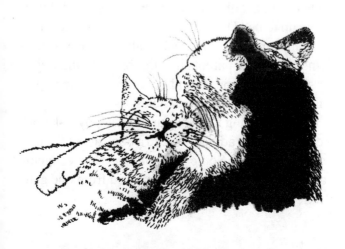

Extreme stress for the mother cat can lead to excessive moving of the kittens, lack of milk production and even neglect or cannibalism.

New Puppy

Q: We have decided to buy a puppy for our son for his birthday. What suggestions do you have for choosing the right dog?

A: Puppies can make wonderful gifts for youngsters who are mature enough to take on the serious responsibility of being a pet owner. It is very important, of course, to be careful about your selection.

Make sure the puppy is healthy and friendly, and think about what he or she will be like as a grown dog. Try to see the puppy's parents, and find out as much as possible about them. Are the mother and father both healthy and friendly? How big did they grow up to be? Do they have medical disorders that the puppy might inherit, such as allergies or hip problems? Have the parents had trouble with their eyes or skin? If so, you should be aware that the puppy might have the same tendencies.

If you are going to buy a purebred puppy, ask your veterinarian for advice, or read a book about the history of the breed. Some types of dogs have congenital medical problems that are passed from one generation to the next.

Mixed-breed puppies can be healthier than pure-breds because of the diversity of their gene pools, which tend to dilute inherited medical disorders. You might consider getting a puppy from the pound. Pound puppies can show extraordinary devotion, as though they realize that they were rescued from a desperate situation. In addition, you get the pleasure of knowing that you personally saved a little creature's life.

Look at the puppy and make sure its eyes are clear and free of matted discharge. Make sure the puppy isn't coughing or sneezing and doesn't have a runny nose. The puppy should have a lot of energy and not be too thin. The skin and hair should look healthy. Also, be sure to find out the puppy's exact age and whether or not it has received the first vaccinations for distemper, parvo and coronavirus.

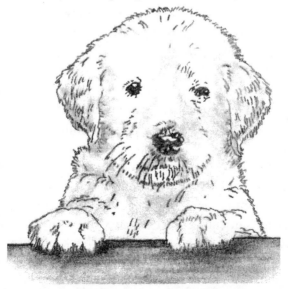

Try to spend some time watching the puppy playing with other dogs, and see how it reacts when it is alone with you. If you have other pets in the family, try to arrange to introduce the puppy to them before making a final decision.

When you think that you have selected just the right puppy, immediately schedule a physical exam with your veterinarian. Be sure to keep the option of returning the puppy if it has major medical problems. Your veterinarian will check the puppy's teeth, ears, eyes, heart, lungs and skin, and give vaccinations and worming medication, as well as advice on nutrition, housebreaking and training.

Nutrition (cats)

Q: My cats eat dog food. It's cheaper and easier to feed all of my pets the same thing, and they seem to like it OK. Now one of my cats is sick. Could it be from the dog food?

A: Cats have very distinct nutritional needs that dog food doesn't satisfy. Serious medical problems can result from feeding your cats nothing but dog food.

Cats need more protein and fat in their diets than dogs. In addition, they cannot manufacture an essential amino acid called taurine. A deficiency of taurine can cause heart disease, infertility and the degeneration of the retina in the back of the eye, resulting in blindness.

Cats also can have nutritional deficiencies from eating poor quality cat food.

All-meat diets or unprescribed calcium and phosphorus supplements can alter the normal calcium/phosphorus ratio and result in the loss of calcium from the cat's bones. This causes fractures and deformities.

Raw fish contains the enzyme thiaminase that destroys the B vitamin thiamine and can result in seizures.

Balanced nutrition is essential for the health of your cat. Only high quality, balanced, all-natural cat foods—either canned, kibble or both—should be fed to cats.

In addition, a food supplement is recommended even if you are feeding your cat the highest quality premium foods. Heat, light and oxygen can destroy the essential oils or fatty acids during the manufacture and storage of commercial pet foods. A deficiency in fatty acids can result in many skin problems, including a dry, scaly skin with excessive shedding, a dull, dry coat and itching. A food supplement containing essential fatty acids, borage oil, marine lipids and lecithin is very important for healthy skin and the best possible hair coat.

A good multiple vitamin also can help provide a long, happy, healthy life.

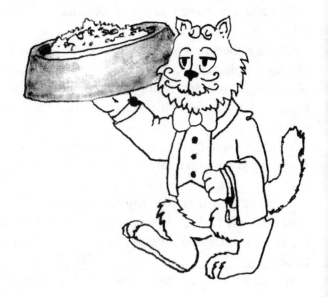

Nutrition (dogs)

Q: What should I feed my dogs? There are so many choices of canned food and kibble in the pet stores and supermarkets, I don't know how to decide which ones are best.

A: Pet foods vary tremendously in quality. Different foods can have exactly the same listed ingredients and percentage of nutrients but big differences in quality. This is due to the digestibility of the food and the extent to which the gastrointestinal tract can absorb the nutrients.

Manufacturers list only the crude protein rather than the amount that your pet actually can use. For example, protein from chicken or eggs is much higher quality and more absorbable than protein from chicken or meat by-products—unwanted parts like chicken feathers or ground up cowhide and hooves.

Dog foods often are loaded with sugar, artificial flavors, colorings and preservatives—especially the semi-moist foods.

Whenever possible, select a dog food with whole meats listed rather than meat by-products. Look for ingredients like chicken, lamb, rice, barley, eggs and acidophilus.

Dogs usually do best on kibble with limited amounts of canned food. The kibble keeps teeth cleaner and healthier than if the dog just ate canned food.

Virtually all commercial pet foods, including the "premium" foods, are heat processed and stored for a period of time before they are sold. Heat processing and exposure to air and light can destroy important nutrients such as essential fatty acids. Therefore, it is critical to add a high-quality cold-processed food supplement that contains additional essential fatty acids. "Essential" refers to the fact that these fatty acids are required by the body for a normal skin and hair coat. However, the body is unable to manufacture fatty acids. In addition to fatty acids, the food supplement should contain marine lipids and borage oil, as well as lecithin for absorbability.

Some pet owners prefer to home-cook meals for their pets. If you choose this course, care should be

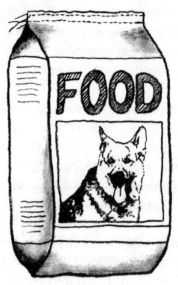

taken to include the necessary nutrients and provide a balanced diet.

Parvovirus

Q: My dog recently got very sick with vomiting and diarrhea. The veterinarian tested him and discovered that he has parvo. How is that possible? He had his shots.

A: Mutations in the potentially deadly and highly contagious parvovirus can result in "breaks" in parvo vaccine coverage. It is possible to develop a milder form of the disease even though your dog has been inoculated.

Other reasons for "breaks" in vaccination coverage include outdated or mishandled vaccines or the possibility that your dog's immune system isn't responding in a normal way.

The rugged parvovirus can survive for months in extreme temperatures and can be carried into a household on someone's shoes. Even if your dog hasn't come
into contact with other animals, the danger of him having been infected with parvovirus exists.

The first signs of parvovirus often are depression, loss of energy and loss of appetite. Vomiting typically develops next, followed by diarrhea and dehydration. The pet's stool has a very bad odor and may be tinged with blood.

The parvovirus affects the immune systems of dogs and lowers the number of white blood cells that fight off the infection. Treatment, which should take place in an isolation ward of a veterinary hospital, consists of giving intravenous fluids and electrolytes, as well as various medications including antibiotics to fight secondary bacterial infections. It is critical to get aggressive treatment as early as possible.

All dogs should be vaccinated for parvo, as well as distemper and coronavirus. Puppies receive their first combination distemper-parvo vaccination at 6 to 8 weeks of age. Boosters should be given at three-week intervals until the puppy is 16 to 19 weeks of age. Many veterinarians recommend that the last vaccination in the series be given at 20 to 24 weeks.

At one year, puppies should have a distemperparvo combination booster. After that, a single distemper-parvo booster every year for the rest of the dog's life is the best way to prevent this potentially fatal disease.

It is very important for all dogs to keep current on these vaccinations. Dogs can be even more susceptible to parvo as they get older because of weakened resistance. Also, parvovirus, like many other viruses, has been able to continue to mutate and change form, increasing the necessity of receiving a booster every year.

Physical Exam

Q: How often should my pets get checkups if they are healthy?

A: A thorough physical examination at least once each year is a very important part of preventive health care for both dogs and cats. Puppies and kittens should be checked as soon as possible after they are born and should begin their routine vaccinations at about eight weeks of age. Some pet owners elect to have their animals checked every six months.

At the start of the physical exam, your veterinarian will take a complete history of your pet's health, including past medical problems, behavior, diet and vaccinations. The animal's temperature, weight, pulse and respiration also will be noted. Using a stethoscope, the veterinarian will listen to the pet's heart to check for any irregular sounds and to the lungs for any unusual noises or breathing rates.

Your pet's eyes can reflect its health, often helping the veterinarian determine quickly if the animal has anemia, jaundice or infection. Using an ophthalmoscope, the veterinarian also will check for corneal lesions, proper pupil size, reaction to light and abnormal bleeding or discharge.

Next, your veterinarian will check your animal's teeth for decay or excessive buildup of tartar. A dentistry may be recommended to keep the teeth strong and healthy—an important part of the digestive process. Your pet's gums, lips, tongue, palate, throat and tonsils also will be examined.

An otoscope will be used to check your pet's ears for wax buildup, foreign bodies or infection. Then your veterinarian will palpate or feel the animal's abdomen, kidneys, liver, intestines and spleen to check for tumors, enlarged organs, gas, fluids or other abnormalities. The reproductive organs, legs, joints, paws and foot pads, neck, tail and spine all should be evaluated, too. A fecal or stool sample will be taken to check for worms.

The skin will be checked for parasites (such as ticks and fleas), tumors, abscesses and infections. The condition of your pet's hair coat can tell a great deal about the animal's nutrition. Hair and skin also can signal problems with the thyroid glands, other hormones, or pollen and food allergies.

In addition, your veterinarian can give advice on the proper shampoo for your pet's individual skin and hair coat needs, recommend how often to bathe and suggest the most effective flea control.

After the routine physical exam, your veterinarian might recommend further diagnostic procedures, such as a blood test, urinalysis, skin scraping, ear swab, electrocardiogram or X-ray.

Poisonous Plants

Q: My grandmother says I shouldn't bring my cat to her house over the holidays because she uses lots of poinsettias for decorations. Are they really harmful?

A: The beautiful red or white poinsettia leaves produce a mild sap that can irritate an animal's skin if touched, and upset the stomach and intestinal tract if eaten. Consult your veterinarian immediately if your cat eats this plant. Any portion of your pet's skin that comes in contact with the sap should be washed thoroughly with soap and water.

Other plants in the poinsettia family include tinsel tree, crown-of-thorns, milk bush, candelilla or snow-on-the-mountain. They also produce a milky sap that irritates the skin and causes inflammation of the lining of the eyelid or irritation of the mouth.

Mistletoe is another plant often used for holiday decorations that can be very dangerous for cats. All parts of the plant are toxic, but the berries are especially poisonous. If eaten, mistletoe can cause nausea, vomiting and diarrhea. This is a medical emergency, and pets should be taken to a veterinarian immediately.

A variety of other plants that often are used around the holidays also could cause problems for your cat. Castor beans, for example, have colorful seeds used for necklaces or festive decorations. The large seeds can be extremely poisonous. Symptoms may not appear for eighteen to twenty-four hours. Then, the body temperature rises and the cat becomes slightly depressed and thirsty. Severe diarrhea and fatal convulsions will follow unless the animal gets emergency treatment immediately.

Another legume popular in jewelry and holiday decoration, the rosary pea, is extremely toxic to cats. The seeds are bright red with a black spot and are used in rosaries or necklaces. The shell of the seed is very hard and difficult to crack, but when strung on a necklace, the poisonous center is exposed. Symptoms usually develop slowly and include a rising temperature, depression and a loss of appetite, followed by violent vomiting. The cat may lose coordination or become paralyzed.

Toxic plants usually are not as serious a problem for dogs as they are for cats. Dogs rarely are fond of eating plants, and usually the most severe problem that results is limited vomiting and diarrhea.

However, dieffenbachia (dumbcane) is a severe threat to both dogs and cats because it causes the throat to swell and can result in suffocation.

Pollen Allergies

Q: Several times every year, my dog chews her front paws and rubs her face constantly. What could be causing that?

A: When and where your pet itches can provide your veterinarian with valuable clues to the cause of the problem. For example, seasonal episodes of itching on the face and paws are typical of allergies to pollens from trees, grasses or weeds.

Pollen allergies are inherited, and usually appear when a pet is between one and three years old.

By contrast, dogs that are allergic to fleas tend to chew their backs above the tail, and dogs with scabies mites itch everywhere—except for the back. Food allergies can result in non-seasonal itching all over the pet's body.

Pets often are allergic to seasonal pollens from such plants as bermuda grass, ragweed and oak trees. Skin testing or blood analysis can identify which pollens cause your pet's allergic reaction.

The best treatment for allergies to pollens or other inhalants such as tobacco, smog, house dust and perfume is simply to avoid exposing your dog to any of the substances that cause the allergies. Daily vacuuming and air filtration systems can be helpful in this effort.

After your pet's allergies are identified through skin testing or blood analysis, antigens can be injected under the skin in increasing amounts to help block the allergic reaction. Your veterinarian can train you to give the injections at home. Surprisingly, most owners find the injections easy to give, and the results can be very rewarding.

Antihistamines can be useful in controlling pollen allergies in pets, but they are generally more effective in treating human allergies because of the respiratory nature of allergy symptoms in people.

Food supplements containing marine lipids (fish oils), borage oil and essential fatty acids can be dramatically effective in controlling pollen allergies. Adding the proper food supplement to your pet's diet often not only stops the itching completely within a month, but can result in a vastly improved hair coat.

Cortisone shots or pills may be recommended by your veterinarian to stop the itch-scratch cycle. The use of these steroids by themselves to treat allergies may be dangerous because they can cause serious side effects.

Pre-surgery Tests

Q: My dog needs some surgery, and our veterinarian has recommended some blood tests before the operation. Why is that necessary?

A: Your dog probably will have a total body function blood test before receiving a general anesthetic for surgery. This is a very important precaution to determine if your animal's organs are functioning properly and if there are any other hidden medical problems.

One part of the blood test consists of getting a complete count of the numbers and types of white and red blood cells. This helps to determine whether your pet is normal and healthy or has underlying problems, such as anemia, possible bacterial or viral infection, allergies, parasites or even cancer.

For example, if your dog is anemic, the number of red blood cells will be low, and they might appear pale under the microscope.

If the immune system is suppressed, the number of certain types of white blood cells can be low. With bacterial infections, the number can be higher than normal. If leukemia is present, large numbers of unusual white blood cells can be seen under the microscope. Allergies and parasites can cause an increase in a specific type of white blood cell, and sometimes microscopic parasites can invade the blood cells, or the cells can change shape or size when various other diseases are present.

Another part of the blood test is called a chemistry panel. Certain chemicals in the blood change if major body organs such as the liver and kidneys aren't working properly.

For example, if your pet has kidney disease, toxins begin to build up in the blood because the kidneys aren't able to filter them properly. Certain levels of chemical enzymes also then build up in the blood if the liver is not functioning properly. Therefore, it is possible to test the function of both the liver and kidneys by measuring these chemicals in the blood.

High blood-sugar levels can indicate a lack of production of insulin by the pancreas, resulting in diabetes. Diabetes can have many complications, such as rapid cataract formation and low immunity to infections.

It is also very important for electrolytes, such as sodium and potassium, to be at proper levels and in balance. Certain diseases greatly change these electrolytes, causing life-threatening situations. Persistent vomiting and diarrhea or hormone imbalance in the adrenal glands can cause an electrolyte imbalance, which would show up on the blood chemistry test.

Pyometra (uterus infection)

Q: My sister's dog died last week from a "pyometra." What exactly is that and how can it be treated and prevented?

A: Pyometra is an infection of the uterus. This condition is a life-threatening medical emergency, especially if bacterial infection is trapped in the uterus because the cervix, or neck of the uterus, is closed.

Pyometras usually occur in middle-aged or older dogs and cats that haven't been spayed. The problem most often starts two to three weeks after a heat cycle.

A pet with pyometra shows a wide variety of symptoms because toxins rapidly build up in its system. The animal often becomes depressed, refuses to eat, suffers from vomiting and diarrhea, wants to drink large quantities of water and urinates more than normal. If the cervix is open, you may notice a yellow or reddish discharge. Sometimes the pet may constantly lick the area, thereby eliminating any signs of discharge.

Pet owners who notice any of these symptoms should get their animals checked immediately by a veterinarian. Emergency action must be taken to prevent kidney damage from the toxins or possible rupture of the uterus which would release pus into the abdomen.

Diagnosis can be made by physical exam, blood test, X-ray, ultrasound and microscopic examination of vaginal discharge. Surgical removal of the ovaries and uterus (ovariohysterectomy) is the usual treatment.

Certain drugs sometimes can be used instead of surgery in the treatment of pyometras in important breeding bitches.

Researchers don't understand all of the factors that cause pyometras, but animals that have never been pregnant, that experience irregular estrous cycles or that have false pregnancies are more likely to develop pyometras as they get older.

The best treatment for a pyometra is prevention. The potential problem can be eliminated by having female dogs or cats spayed before one year of age. This surgery also dramatically decreases the chances that the pet ever will have breast cancer.

Rabies Vaccination

Q: How often does the law require my dog to be vaccinated against rabies?

A: Ideally, young dogs should be vaccinated for rabies at three months of age, then receive a rabies booster vaccination when they are one year old.

Typically, dogs over the age of one year are required to be vaccinated for rabies every three years, although local regulations may vary. Veterinarians usually recommend that puppies be vaccinated for rabies as soon after three months of age as possible. The rabies vaccine is required for your dog by law because an outbreak of rabies could be deadly for humans, as well as animals.

A rabies certificate is required for interstate travel in the United States, and many countries around the world have strict regulations to control the spread of this dangerous health threat.

Although the DHLP-P (distemper-parvo combination) vaccination usually is not required by law like the rabies vaccination, it may be even more critical to your dog's health because the DHLP-P vaccination can prevent several more common potentially life-threatening infectious diseases.

Rat Poison

Q: My neighbors have rats in their garage, and they are planning to put out rat poison. I'm afraid my dog might get into it. Would that be dangerous?

A: Rat poison is very dangerous for any pet. If warfarin or similar chemicals are eaten, they often can be fatal.

The poison is tempting to most animals because it has a sweet taste intended to attract the rats.

Poisons of this type interfere with vitamin K in an animal's body and prevent the normal blood clotting process.

Symptoms of rat poisoning can appear two to five days after the initial exposure. Because the animal's blood is not clotting properly, you may notice blood in the stool or urine, or coming from the nose or mouth. The whites of your pet's eyes or the skin may have red areas due to hemorrhaging. Much of the bleeding can be inside, so you might not notice the problem right away.

Sometimes the first sign of this kind of poisoning is difficulty in breathing because of bleeding in the chest. Blood loss and hemorrhaging can cause anemia, weakness, pale gums and shock.

A pet that has eaten rat poison should be hospitalized immediately. For the first few hours after the poison has been swallowed, your veterinarian can induce vomiting, then follow up quickly with appropriate treatment. If it is too late to induce vomiting, your veterinarian will take blood tests to help gauge the severity of any internal bleeding caused by the poison.

Vitamin K is given to correct the clotting defect. The chest or abdomen may need to be drained of blood, and X-rays often are necessary to determine the extent of internal bleeding. Blood transfusions and treatment for shock also may be required.

Ringworm

Q: Our kitten has little areas on her face and ears where the hair is falling out, and the skin looks dry and scaly. Now my son has red patches on his arms and hands. What could be causing that?

A: Your kitten—and your son—could have ringworm. This common fungus (not a "worm" at all) is easily transmitted from pets to people, especially to children.

Your kitten should be examined and treated by a veterinarian. The most accurate way to diagnose ringworm is by microscopic examination of the hair and skin or by growing the fungus in a special culture bottle.

Depending on the extent of the infection, your kitten will be treated with a series of anti-fungal baths, appropriate creams and ointments, and possibly even oral medication in severe cases. In addition, the environment should be thoroughly cleaned to prevent reinfection. It usually takes four to six weeks to clear up ringworm.

Be sure to consult a physician about the patches on your son's skin.

Scabies Mites

Q: I have two dogs that itch constantly. They don't have fleas, but they rub, chew and scratch their ears, elbows and stomachs all the time. What could be wrong?

A: The itchiest skin problem that a dog can have is caused by a type of mange called scarcoptic mange or scabies. Your dogs have symptoms that are typical for this condition.

Scabies is caused by a small mite that is easily transferred from one dog to another by direct contact. Perhaps one of your dogs picked up scabies mites at your groomer's, your boarding kennel, your veterinary clinic or while playing in the park with other neighborhood dogs.

Dogs with scabies often scratch so much that hair comes out in chunks, and the skin becomes crusty, scaly and infected. The itch is so persistent that a dog may prefer to scratch instead of eating or sleeping.

Scabies often makes dogs smell like rancid oil. Usually the ears, elbows and stomach are the most dramatically affected areas. The back of the dog rarely itches, helping to distinguish scabies from several other skin conditions.

However, if a dog has flea allergies in addition to scabies, the animal's whole body can itch, further complicating the diagnosis.

Scabies mites are very difficult to find. A skin

scraping is taken from the scaly, dry areas on the elbows and ears. These scales are examined for the mites under a microscope. Since these mites are rarely found, many times the skin problem is diagnosed from the symptoms and the response to treatment rather than from actually identifying a scabies mite.

Treatment consists of killing the mites with special medications, fighting the skin infection with antibiotics, soothing the sore skin with shampoos and coat conditioners, and reducing the itching with anti-inflammatory drugs. Also, your dogs' home environment must be cleaned thoroughly with a disinfectant.

Dogs with scabies mites usually respond very well to treatment within a couple of weeks.

People can get scabies from dogs, but the itching is only temporary because the mites will not reproduce on human skin.

Scratched Eyes

Q: My dog was scratched in the eye by our new kitten. Now she is squinting and her eye is red. There also is some discharge. What should I do?

A: Cat scratches are a common injury for dogs. Scratches to the eye can result in damage to the cornea or surface layer of the eye.

The cornea has many nerves and, as a result, is extremely sensitive. When the cornea is traumatized, it can be very painful and often results in tearing and squinting. Sometimes the third eyelid covers the damaged area as the animal's body tries to protect the wound. Your dog also might constantly rub the eye in an effort to relieve the discomfort.

The injury to the cornea may be too small to even see, but any damage to the eye should be immediately examined by a veterinarian.

A special dye can be put into the eye and then examined under a light to reveal any areas that are damaged or ulcerated. If the injury is deep or there is debris or a foreign body in the eye, surgical correction under anesthesia will be necessary. If the laceration goes through the cornea, very fine stitches may be used to repair the wound.

In some cases, a veterinarian might temporarily suture the eyelids together or create a protective flap using the third eyelid to allow healing. Sometimes even soft contact lenses can be used to protect an ulcer in your pet's eye.

Ulcers and wounds to the cornea can become increasingly larger and may become infected. If there is bleeding, the wound is very deep and should be treated as a serious medical emergency.

In addition to wounds, some dogs develop corneal ulcers because of a lack of tear production. Your veterinarian can measure the amount of tears that your dog produces to determine if an artificial tear solution should be prescribed.

Never treat eye injuries yourself. The use of eye ointments containing cortisone can be very dangerous if there is any kind of laceration or ulceration of the eye.

Seborrhea

Q: My cocker spaniel has oily, scaly, itchy skin that has a bad odor. What do you suggest to treat that problem?

A: The symptoms that you describe are typical of various skin problems, but seborrhea is a chronic disease that is especially widespread among cocker spaniels. Seborrhea is often secondary to other skin problems such as allergies, hormone imbalances and bacterial infections.

Itching often accompanies the scaly dandruff, and the scratching that results can cause "hot spots" and other areas of soreness and infection.

Seborrhea usually is controlled by treating any underlying cause such as low thyroid function or allergies, and by using special medicated shampoos and soothing coat conditioners.

However, researchers have found that large daily oral doses of vitamin A can have excellent results. Cocker spaniels with seborrhea often show remarkable improvement within three weeks and can be completely cured within two or three months.

The dosage of vitamin A should be carefully

monitored by a veterinarian to guard against possible side effects. Excessive doses of vitamin A can be very toxic.

Seborrhea that affects cocker spaniels, as well as other breeds, is like seborrhea in humans, although it cannot be transmitted between pet and owner.

Many other skin problems show symptoms similar to those you describe. A veterinarian can examine your pet to rule out hypothyroidism, pollen allergies, food allergies, scabies, flea allergies or other causes of scaling, itching and odor.

Senior Pets

Q: What can I do to help my dear little sixteen-year-old dog live longer? She still is in pretty good health, but I know she doesn't have as much energy as she used to.

A: Your "senior citizen" pet already has lived a very full life. Regular checkups by a veterinarian can help make sure that she continues to stay in good health and that any medical problems which might develop in the coming years are treated promptly.

With some variance relating to breed, many dogs begin experiencing the changes of advancing age starting around the time they are eight years old. Large breeds begin to age sooner than small breeds.

Two types of changes affect older pets with increasing frequency. First, age-related changes in vision and hearing are normal and develop in most animals. Second, diseases such as cancer, arthritis, diabetes and heart, liver or kidney problems become more prevalent as pets age. Most of the medical problems in this second category can be treated if diagnosed early.

In addition to annual checkups, vaccinations and dentistries, many veterinarians offer a complete geriatric checkup for your older pet. In addition to the physical exam, several diagnostic tests can identify areas where any medical problems might be developing.

X-rays can help uncover changes such as enlargements or reductions in organ size, accumulation of fluid, presence of tumors, arthritic changes in joints, and the presence of bladder stones.

An electrocardiogram (ECG) can help your veterinarian assess your pet's heart and detect any irregular, slow or weak heartbeat.

A urinalysis gives an indication of how the kidneys are functioning and also serves as an all-purpose screen for systemic disease.

A complete blood count (CBC) can help in the diagnosis of bacterial and viral infections, anemia and clotting problems.

A blood chemistry panel indicates abnormalities in blood sugar levels, and liver or kidney function.

Consultation about a diet that meets your pet's changing nutritional needs also is an important part of any geriatric checkup. As pets get older, their nutritional needs begin to differ from those of younger animals.

For example, older pets should have less protein in their diets, and their vitamin and mineral requirements generally increase. Fewer calories are usually necessary because they are not as active as when they were younger.

Skin Care Products

Q: Dr. Thomas, I know that you have developed all-natural skin care products for dogs and cats that are used all over the world. Why are your products the best?

A: I originally formulated the all-natural Veterinarian's Best skin care products for my own dermatology patients at the Southern California Veterinary Hospital & Animal Skin Clinic.

I was frustrated with all of the chemicals that are used in pet shampoos and flea control products, as well as the extensive use of potentially dangerous steroids and cortisone in treating allergies in dogs and cats.

As an alternative, I developed the Veterinarian's Best Hypoallergenic Shampoo, Hot Spot Shampoo, Moisturizing Conditioner, Hot Spot Spray and Vita-Derm food supplement. These products contain human cosmetic-grade ingredients, rather than the chemical-grade ingredients found in most other pet products. In addition, they contain very special ingredients like the Australian tea tree oil, borage oil, aloe vera, chamomile, vitamins A and E, and marine lipids with omega 3.

In studies at university veterinary medical dermatology departments, the Veterinarian's Best products were found to be extremely effective in treating pets with severe skin problems, and achieved excellent results in providing relief for dogs that could no longer take steroids or cortisone to control itching caused by pollen allergies.

• **Veterinarian's Best Vita-Derm** food supplement for dogs and cats adds marine lipids with omega 3 and essential fatty acids, borage oil, lecithin, and vitamins A and E to your pet's diet each day to promote beautiful, healthy skin and hair coat.

Essential fatty acids are nutrients which are important for health and cannot be manufactured in the body. Fatty acids are very sensitive to heat, and as a result they are destroyed in pet foods during the manufacturing process and later when pet foods are stored. Vita-Derm is a source of cold-processed essential fatty acids which ensures that nutrition is preserved.

In addition, lecithin helps the body absorb essential fatty acids, and vitamin E helps keep them from oxidizing and being destroyed. Vitamins A and E, and borage oil help heal damaged skin. Both marine lipids (fish oils) and borage oil in Vita-Derm help eliminate itching caused by pollen allergies.

These essential fatty acids, vitamins and marine lipids are very important for normal skin and hair, too. They also help to eliminate itching, excessive shedding and dry, flaky dandruff.

• **Veterinarian's Best Hot Spot Spray** gives dogs and cats immediate relief from flea allergy dermatitis, "hot spots," sores, red welts, and itching caused by fleas and allergies. This remarkable spray contains tea tree oil, used for centuries by Australian aborigines to heal wounds and repel fleas and mosquitoes. Hot Spot Spray can be used as often as needed for healing or to control fleas. Hot Spot Spray can be combined with Veterinarian's Best Shampoo for a natural flea shampoo, or mixed with the Moisturizing Conditioner to make a natural flea dip.

• **Veterinarian's Best Moisturizing Conditioner** is specifically formulated to penetrate and revitalize your pet's skin and hair coat while adding body and a healthy, shining luster. Natural healing and moisturizing ingredients help to eliminate itching, dryness and dandruff.

This conditioner is ideal for the normal coat which needs more body and luster, and also is very valuable in treating many skin problems. It can be used after every bath as a moisturizer which is left on the coat to soothe and protect, and it can be sprayed lightly over the entire hair coat daily or when brushing. It is not oily or greasy, and gives your pet's coat a fresh, pleasant smell.

• **Veterinarian's Best Shampoos** are scientifically formulated to gently and thoroughly cleanse your pet's hair coat without harsh soap while adding moisture and body. A special combination of natural and rejuvenating ingredients helps to eliminate itching and rough, scaly, irritated or dry skin. Hot Spot Shampoo adds Australian tea tree oil for pets that suffer from flea allergy dermatitis and various skin infections. The Hypoallergenic Shampoo is designed for normal to dry skin and is particularly good for top show coats and the sensitive skin of puppies and kittens.

These shampoos are perfect for keeping normal hair soft, healthy and shiny, as well as for use in conjunction with a veterinarian's prescribed treatment for skin problems. They are designed to cleanse infected areas, soothe red, sore, itchy skin and reduce dandruff by moisturizing and removing dead skin.

Veterinarian's Best skin care products can be used individually or in combination with each other. For best results, use all of the products together as a team the way they were designed.

Veterinarian's Best skin care products are carried in pet stores throughout the world.

For more information about Veterinarian's Best all-natural skin care products, write:

Veterinarian's Best
P.O. Box 4459, Dept. B
Santa Barbara, CA 93103

Spay and Neuter

Q: When do you recommend that dogs and cats be spayed or neutered? Will this change their personalities?

A: Dogs and cats can be spayed or neutered as early as six months of age, although many veterinarians prefer to wait to neuter male cats until they are about seven to nine months old.

The main purpose for spaying and neutering animals, of course, is to prevent unwanted pregnancies. Many of the homeless puppies and kittens from these accidental litters suffer neglect and eventually are destroyed.

Neutering male dogs and cats also can help prevent unwanted roaming and fighting. Sometimes this can make a pet more affectionate to the owner and much easier to live with. In addition, the surgery reduces the risk of prostate disease and various types of tumors.

Female dogs or cats will be healthier and look better without unwanted puppies or kittens. Spaying females when they are under one year of age will dramatically reduce the chances of breast cancer later in life.

Female dogs and cats that have not been spayed are at risk of developing pyometra, a life-threatening medical emergency where the uterus becomes infected. Any change in your pet's personality after being altered will be from the natural maturing process, rather than a result of the surgery. Another concern is that the pet might gain weight. After being altered, some animals need fewer calories. The amount of food they receive should be adjusted by the owner depending on the level of activity and rate of metabolism. A male dog that is fighting and carousing needs more calories than after he is neutered, when he is content to stay closer to home.

For both spay and neuter surgeries, a general anesthesia is used. Your veterinarian will advise you about the importance of a pre-anesthesia blood test, depending on the age and health of your pet. This test can help determine how safe the surgery will be for your pet and sometimes indicates the need for using a special anesthetic.

To help avoid complications in your pet's spay or neuter surgery, make sure that the operation will be performed in a sterile surgery room by a licensed veterinarian.

After surgery, most veterinarians prefer to have patients recover overnight at the hospital, except for some male cats that might be sent home the same day.

Steroids

Q: My veterinarian keeps giving my dog cortisone shots about every three weeks to control itching. I'm worried about side

effects. What should I do?

A: Cortisone is a steroid drug well known and widely used as an anti-inflammatory. Cortisone is essential in the treatment of many cancers and autoimmune diseases and can be effective in controlling itching caused by certain allergies.

However, cortisone provides only temporary relief for itching—and there can be some very serious side effects.

Stopping the itch without cortisone should be the goal of every pet owner, but unfortunately these steroids often are grossly overused.

Cortisone affects the entire body, including muscles, skin, liver, kidneys and the thyroid. It suppresses the immune system so the body is less able to fight off infections and disease. A common side effect is increased urination.

Animals that are given steroids too often or in inappropriately high doses can develop the iatrogenic ("doctor-caused") Cushing's disease.

Dogs that suffer from Cushing's disease often have increased appetite, increased water consumption and increased urination. Their abdomens can become swollen, their livers enlarged, and they often have symmetrical hair loss. Their coats usually become very dry and thin, their skin becomes thin and bruises easily, and they are susceptible to skin infections. Dogs with Cushing's also suffer from thinning muscle tissue and depression. If not diagnosed early, the disease can be fatal.

There are several effective alternatives to the use of cortisone and steroids in treating itching.

Food supplements that provide essential fatty acids with borage oil, marine lipids (fish oils) and lecithin can provide dramatic results in just a few weeks. Any one of these ingredients alone is not as effective as using them in combination.

Antihistamines can help reduce itching related to allergic reactions. They work best when combined with the proper food supplement.

Topical anti-inflammatory ingredients such as Australian tea tree oil, aloe vera and chamomile in the form of sprays or shampoos can have a soothing effect that immediately relieves itching. Topical anesthetics such as lidocaine and hydrocortisone can dry, burn and further damage the skin. Imagine putting alcohol on an open wound on your own skin!

The combination of tea tree oil, aloe vera and chamomile not only relieves the itching, redness and pain, but has the additional benefits of being antiseptic, anti-fungal and antibacterial.

Probably the most effective approach to eliminating the need for steroids in controlling itching has been a program tested in both university and private clinical trials which combines a food supplement (containing marine lipids, essential fatty acids and borage oil) with all-natural topical shampoos, sprays and conditioners (containing tea tree oil, chamomile and aloe vera). Always avoid chemical dips, sprays and shampoos that actually can increase your pet's itching and discomfort. (See *Skin*

Care Products.)
Stings

Q: My dog keeps getting stung by wasps in our yard. I see him jumping and biting at them, and every so often he gets puffy red areas on his face. Is that dangerous?

A: Dogs and cats are more likely than humans to be bitten or stung by spiders, bees, wasps, ants and snakes because pets like to play with these interesting little creatures. The results can be painful—and potentially dangerous.

Initial symptoms of bites and stings are swelling and redness, often in the face area, and these signs usually start within an hour. Later the symptoms can include pain in the muscles and joints, vomiting, diarrhea, becoming uncoordinated or paralyzed, or even going into convulsions. The site of the bite or sting also can become ulcerated.

Dogs like to try to catch bees with their mouths, and the result often is a painful sting. Common spiders with poisonous bites include the black widow spider and the brown recluse spider. Reactions to stings and snake bites are more likely than spider bites to result in shock.

Treatment for bites and stings includes keeping the animal calm and applying cold packs to reduce swelling. If the reaction is severe or the pet is in shock, be sure to get immediate medical attention from your veterinarian. Antihistamines and steroids can help reduce the inflammation and tissue reaction. In severe cases, epinephrine and fluids also are given to help counteract shock.

Bites and stings can cause such severe damage to the tissue that it begins to die and often becomes infected. This can cause the wound to heal slowly.

Each exposure to a bite or sting can cause a reaction that is more severe than the time before. Help keep your pet safe by thoroughly spraying your yard to eliminate the wasps, as well as other stinging insects, including ants.

Talking to Your Cat

Q: My friend says that she actually can "talk" with her cat. Is that possible or is she just a little nutty?

A: Cats communicate using vocal sounds, body positions and by marking territories with different body odors. Many of your cat's signals can be learned and interpreted by people, making communication between cats and humans more extensive than between humans and other species.

Purring is a common form of communication. Cats often purr when happy or having a pleasurable experience, and a prolonged purr is used as a friendly greeting, or a request for food or attention. Cats also can purr when extremely ill or dying. This might be a way of comforting themselves, or it might reflect a state of euphoria.

Demands, complaints and anger are expressed with growls, snarls, hissing, screams and other vocalizations. Calling or crying is used by the female and male to indicate that they are ready to mate. Siamese cats usually are quite loud and expressive. They use different vowel sounds, which are inherited on the same gene that carries their distinctive coat and eye colors.

Your cat will assume different postures, depending on whether it intends to be offensive, defensive or submissive.

In an offensive posture, pupils are constricted and your cat looks its enemy directly in the eyes. Your cat's body is straight and whiskers are forward, indicating intention to attack. The tip of the tail may flag back and forth, showing irritation.

In a defensive posture, your cat's back is arched with hair standing on end. Your cat stands with its side to the enemy to look larger and therefore like more of a threat. Ears are flat, whiskers are back, the nose is wrinkled and teeth may be showing. Tail twitching increases as your cat becomes more and more excited.

In the submissive posture, your cat crouches and may roll over on its side.

Tomcat Spraying

Q: My tomcat has suddenly started spraying urine on my furniture. He never did this before. What causes this awful behavior?

A: The type of spraying that you describe could be caused either by a behavior problem or a medical problem—such as a urinary infection, bladder problem or even a hormonal imbalance.

It is important to take your cat to a veterinarian for a complete physical examination to make sure there isn't a medical reason for the inappropriate behavior. Neutering can help to eliminate spraying tendencies—and the related need for territorial roaming and fighting—especially in young tomcats before the habit is firmly ingrained. Neutering also usually makes the odor of urine less offensive.

If the veterinarian gives your pet a clean bill of health, you will need to deal with the spraying as a behavior problem. First, remove your cat from the area being soiled. Then, clean the area well because the odor of urine could encourage a repeat incident. Don't use any products containing ammonia because the urine smell will be enhanced. Enzyme solutions can be especially useful to neutralize odors. Using mothballs or placing your cat's feeding bowl in the area also can help to discourage spraying.

Retrain your cat by keeping him in a small area that contains only a bed, food and litter box. Cats are fastidious by nature and often prefer to go to the toilet in a clean but inappropriate place rather than a messy litter box. Make sure that the litter box is large enough, is in a quiet place and is not being used by too many other cats.

Find a brand of cat litter that your pet likes, and then try not to change it. Some litter odors may be offensive to your cat. Clumping litters usually remain much cleaner.

Of course, be sure to correct any problems that might have prompted the behavior. Often such things as family conflict, a visitor, death of someone in the household, overcrowding or even loneliness can create anxiety and have a strong influence on a cat's personality.

In some extreme cases, medication may be needed to alter behavior.

Toxoplasmosis

Q: I'm pregnant and have four cats. My doctor has expressed a concern about exposure to toxoplasmosis. What are your recommendations as a veterinarian?

A: Toxoplasmosis is a highly infectious disease, sometimes carried by cats, which presents a problem for pregnant women because it can cause birth defects, spontaneous abortion or stillbirth.

Toxoplasmosis is caused by a microscopic intestinal parasite. Cats get the disease by coming in contact with the feces of other cats that are infected or by eating infected raw meat—often rodents or birds. The parasite then can be transferred to humans if they come in contact with infected feces, most commonly when cleaning the litter box or working in a garden.

Most infected cats either show no symptoms at all or give a very mild indication that they don't feel well. A few cats, however, develop sudden, severe signs, including fever, depression, weight loss, coughing, vomiting, diarrhea or lymph nodes that are swollen.

A veterinarian can diagnose toxoplasmosis in cats by examining the feces under a microscope to find eggs of the parasites. Blood tests also can show high levels of antibodies in the blood or other changes in the biochemical values of the internal organs involved.

Sulfa drugs and supportive care are used to treat toxoplasmosis in cats. If a cat shows signs of central nervous system involvement, such as blindness, convulsions or lack of coordination, the chances of survival are poor, and the cat usually dies within three to twelve days. Less severely infected cats usually develop a strong immunity and recover with proper treatment.

To keep your cats from getting toxoplasmosis, discourage them from hunting for birds and rodents, and feed them only commercially prepared cat food or thoroughly cooked meat—never raw meat. Also, make sure your cat's litter box is kept very clean.

Pregnant women should never, never clean litter

boxes themselves. They also should wear gloves when gardening if cats have been around, and always wash their hands after handling cats.

Travel Tips

Q: I am going to take my dog with me on the airplane when I visit my family this year. How can I make sure she is safe?

A: If your dog is small and mild tempered, many airlines will allow you to take her with you in the cabin. Your pet must not create any kind of disturbance and must travel in a standard animal carrying case that fits under the seat.

Before the trip, be sure to take your dog to a veterinarian for a thorough checkup, an update on any vaccinations and a health certificate. It is important to take these health records with you.

Your veterinarian may recommend appropriate tranquilizers for your pet, either to be given before the strange experience of air travel, or at least to take along just in case she becomes upset.

In planning your trip, try to book a direct flight and avoid any connecting flights so you won't have to deal with awkward layovers. If your pet must travel in the airplane's luggage compartment, a missed connection or lost baggage could be disastrous. Also, avoid the busiest travel times so that airport personnel will be available to give more personal attention to you and your pet.Make sure your pet is wearing a collar with an ID tag firmly attached. The tag must have your name, your pet's name, your address and telephone number. Also, make sure your dog has an up-to-date rabies tag.

A strong, comfortable leash is a must for any dog that travels.

Don't feed your pet for about six hours before the trip. Make sure the carrying case has a water tray that is accessible from the outside so that water can be added during the trip if necessary. Be sure to give your pet fresh water just before the trip and as soon as you arrive at your destination.

If your pet must travel in the airplane's luggage compartment, please follow these common sense guidelines:

• Use airlines that hand carry your pet's cage to and from the aircraft, rather than transporting it on a conveyer belt.

• Be sure the cage has strong walls that are water-proof, and sturdy handles so they won't come off during the baggage handling process.

• Be sure the cage has good ventilation on at least three sides and an absorptive covering on the bottom.

• Be sure the cage has a label permanently attached that contains the same information as the dog's tag.

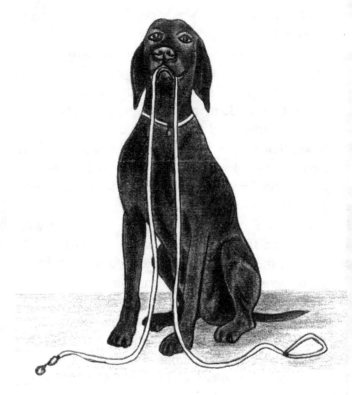

Upset Stomach

Q : My dog is the terror of the neighborhood when it comes to raiding garbage cans. During the past few days he seems to have an upset stomach. Should I be worried?
A: Your pet sounds like a prime candidate for gastroenteritis, an inflammation of the stomach and intestines that can be caused by eating spoiled garbage which is contaminated with bacteria and mold. Also, non-food items such as bones and plastic in

the trash can irritate or tear the lining of the digestive tract.

The most common symptoms of gastroenteritis are vomiting and diarrhea. Other signs include belching and increased water consumption. Some dogs also eat such odd items as dirt, plants or grass.

The diarrhea and vomited material may contain blood that results from increased irritation of the gastrointestinal system. The pet may have an extremely tender abdomen and become dehydrated as a result of vomiting or diarrhea.

Young animals tend to have more problems with eating non-food items from garbage cans, possibly because they are generally more curious, and they have a strong urge to chew on things.

Common dangers from the trash can include cleaning agents, food wrappers and drugs such as aspirin. Other causes of gastroenteritis include hair that accumulates in the stomachs of long-haired cats and dogs, certain types of plants and plant toxins, some bacteria or viruses, and internal parasites such as hookworms and roundworms. Gastroenteritis also can result from diseases of the kidney, liver and pancreas, food allergies, ulcers, cancer or even stress.

Diagnosis of gastroenteritis sometimes is difficult because the causes are so varied. In addition to a physical exam, a veterinarian may need to take abdominal X rays, possibly using a contrast dye to show any abnormalities in the abdomen. A blood sample also can help determine if there are other diseases present. Examination of a stool sample may reveal the presence of intestinal parasites.

In some cases, internal examination with an endoscope or perhaps even exploratory surgery to take a biopsy or remove a foreign object may be necessary.

Treatment of gastroenteritis varies. If your pet seems happy and continues to be hungry, the problem may be minor. Often a bland diet of chicken soup for a few days will be all that is needed to relieve the irritation.

In more serious cases, your pet may not be allowed to eat or drink for several days, and medication to suppress vomiting and slow the movement of ingested materials through the gastrointestinal tract may be appropriate. One danger is dehydration, so your veterinarian may recommend that fluids and electrolytes be administered.

Solid food usually is introduced gradually over several days in the form of a bland diet, or a hypoallergenic diet may be appropriate if a food allergy has caused the problem.

Vaccinations (cats)

Q: Which vaccinations are most important for cats? Do   out-door cats and indoor cats need different kinds of vaccinations?

A: All cats should have two critical laboratory

tests and four very important vaccinations to protect them from deadly diseases.

The tests are for feline leukemia virus (FeLV) and feline AIDS (FIV). Cats that test positive for either disease are very contagious and should be kept away from all other cats.

Although the tests are generally quite accurate, there can be false positive results. In addition, cats that have tested positive for FeLV sometimes can go into remission. Therefore, re-testing of cats for FeLV from time to time is recommended.

Follow your veterinarian's advice about a vaccination schedule. The best timing of vaccinations will vary slightly depending on which brand of vaccine is used.

While there is no vaccination yet for feline AIDS, the FeLV and feline infectious peritonitis (FIP) vaccinations should be given to kittens starting at about eight to ten weeks of age. Boosters then should be given at intervals of two or three weeks until the recommended dosage has been given. Adult cats that are being vaccinated for the first time will get the initial injection, then receive a booster two or three weeks later.

FeLV and FIP boosters should be given every year. The FeLV and FIP vaccinations have no effect on cats already infected with the viruses.

The feline distemper vaccination (FVR-CP) is a combination of inoculations against viral rhinotracheitis, calici and panleukopenia. Kittens should be vaccinated at about eight to ten weeks of age, then receive a booster every three weeks until they are sixteen weeks old. If an adult cat hasn't been vaccinated, then initially two FVR-CP injections are given about two or three weeks apart.

Annual boosters are very important.

Kittens should be vaccinated against rabies at three months of age. Boosters are given one year later, then every one to three years, depending on the vaccine manufacturer's recommendation. All cats that ever go outdoors should be vaccinated against rabies. Indoor cats can benefit from the protection of a rabies vaccination if they happen to accidentally get out of the house and are bitten in a fight with a wild animal.

Cat owners sometimes tend to be less consistent than dog owners in keeping their pets vaccinated, perhaps because cats seem to be so independent.

Vaccinations (dogs)

Q: What vaccinations do you recommend for dogs? I have a new puppy, and I want to be sure that he gets all of his vaccinations when he needs them.

A: Vaccination schedules can vary slightly, depending on the type of inoculation being used and the latest veterinary research. Most veterinarians would concur with the following:

Puppies should be vaccinated at 8, 11 and 17 weeks of age for distemper, hepatitis, leptospirosis, parainfluenza and parvovirus. This usually is given in a single combination injection called DHLP-P. Annual boosters are extremely important.

If an adult dog has not received a DHLP-P inoculation, initially two vaccinations should be given three weeks apart. Because of new outbreaks of parvo from time to time, an additional parvo, booster is recommended at twenty weeks of age.

Rottweilers and Dobermans are especially sensitive to parvo and should receive parvo boosters every six months for the first two years.

Rabies vaccinations, which are required by law, should be given to puppies at four to six months of age. Boosters are given a year later, then every three years. If an adult dog has never been vaccinated against rabies, initially only one vaccination should be given every three years.

Bordetella, which protects against "kennel cough" and similar respiratory infections, is required by most kennels before a dog can be boarded. Puppies usually are given an internasal bordetella vaccination at eight to sixteen weeks of age. Annual internasal boosters are recommended. If the dog is exposed to a kennel situation, or routinely comes in contact with other dogs at a grooming parlor, veterinary clinic, park or in the neighborhood, boosters should be given every six months.

Coronavirus vaccinations are given to puppies at

8, 11, 14 and 17 weeks of age. Annual boosters are recommended. If an adult dog hasn't been vaccinated against the coronavirus, initially two vaccinations are given two or three weeks apart.

Vaccinations are probably the single most important part of your dog's health care. Nothing is more tragic than a wonderful, loyal pet coming down with a deadly disease that was preventable if the owner had only kept the pet current on vaccinations.

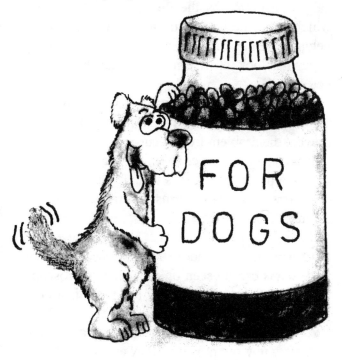

Such fecal exams should be done routinely at least once a year throughout your pet's life, starting at about two or three weeks of age.

Roundworms are quite common in puppies. They can be passed from the mother to the pup through the placenta, and often cause a bloated abdomen and diarrhea. Hookworms and whipworms also can cause dangerous intestinal problems in puppies. All of these parasites should be eliminated with appropriate medication prescribed by a veterinarian as soon as possible.

Tapeworms, another common parasite, are typically transmitted by the flea. Pets swallow fleas, which carry the tapeworm larvae, which then develop inside the animals. Little white tapeworm segments that look like rice sometimes can be seen in a pet's stool.

An injection or pill medication will dissolve the tapeworms, and a good flea control program can prevent the problem from recurring.

If medication is given to kill the tapeworms, but your puppy continues to swallow fleas when she licks herself, the tapeworms will return again and again.

Other internal parasites that can cause severe intestinal problems include giardia and coccidia. These protozoans can be seen only under a microscope. Giardia and coccidia usually are passed through contaminated food or water.

Puppies with any of these internal parasites may have very few symptoms, or they may be very sick, depending on the type of parasite and the extent of the infestation. Often puppies with parasites will have the type of swollen abdomen that you describe, and often they develop diarrhea. Other signs might include a poor hair coat and a lack of appetite.

Unfortunately, many over-the-counter worming remedies are not effective. Your veterinarian can prescribe medication to eliminate the specific parasite and administer it to your puppy in the proper dosage for your pet's age, weight and breed.

About the authors—

Dawn Curie Thomas, DVM, owns the Southern California Veterinary Hospital & Animal Skin Clinic in Los Angeles. She is a 1981 graduate of the University of California, Davis, School of Veterinary Medicine, and a member of the American Academy of Veterinary Dermatology. Dr. Thomas has been a columnist for *The Los Angeles Daily News* and *The Los Angeles Times* and has been featured in *SELF* magazine. In 1989, she developed the Veterinarian's Best line of all-natural, premium-quality skin care products for dogs and cats. The products, originally designed to treat her own dermatology patients without harsh chemicals and dangerous steroids, are now available throughout the world.

William S. Thomas, former newspaper editor and university professor of journalism, holds a masters degree in communications from UCLA. Thomas has worked in various editing capacities for Gannett Newspapers, Times-Mirror, McClatchy Newspapers and Hagadone Newspapers. He has been awarded the DuMont Fellowship and the Gannett Teaching Fellowship.